Beating
Diabetes

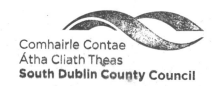

Comhairle Contae
Átha Cliath Theas
South Dublin County Council

CONSULTANTS

Diabetes consultant
Rosie Walker RN BSc (Hons) MA (Ed)
Consultant dietitian
Christopher Cheyette MSc BSc (Hons) RD
Advanced Clinical Specialist Dietitian

Published by The Reader's Digest Association Limited
LONDON • NEW YORK • SYDNEY • MONTREAL

Beating Diabetes

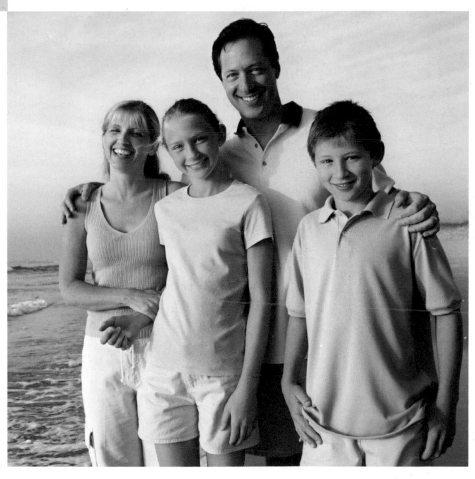

**Hundreds of everyday tips to combat the
disorder and transform your health**

Contents

Beat diabetes in every corner of your life

You do hundreds, even thousands, of things every day, from drinking your morning coffee to turning on the computer to humming a song. Many of them you don't even think about – they're just 'what you do'. Could you change a few of them without affecting your overall day? Of course you could. And what if some of those changes offered the promise of significantly improving your health? Even better.

With that thought in mind, we have put together what may be the most comprehensive menu ever of small changes for better diabetes management. Each tip on the pages ahead is designed to help you to feel great throughout the day, gain better control of your blood glucose, and protect your whole body from the damage that uncontrolled diabetes can cause.

Diabetes isn't a disease that can be treated and forgotten; you take it with you everywhere you go. On the plus side, you can fight it and improve your overall health, no matter where you are. We've created this book to help you to beat your diabetes in every place in your life – your kitchen, your living room, your garden, your neighbourhood, your mind and more. Because it's the little things you do between dawn and dusk that make the difference between getting on top of this common disease or letting it get the better of you.

This book is intended mainly for people with Type 2 diabetes. If you're reading it now, you're already ahead of the game because you're willing to try a few of our 'everyday tips … to transform your health,' as it says on the cover. These ideas are really simple – some take mere minutes to carry out – and you might even enjoy making a few tweaks to your daily routine, just as people enjoy writing with a new pen or wearing a new pair of shoes. If you follow even five or 10 of these clever suggestions regularly, you'll have made huge strides towards improving your health. Incorporate more over the course of time and you'll be surprised and delighted with what happens to your weight, your blood glucose levels, your energy and your sense of well-being.

I should mention that just as you're different from everyone else, so is your diabetes different from everyone else's. These tips are appropriate for just about everyone, but work with your health professionals – your GP, diabetes nurses, registered dietitian and others – to fit them into treatment plans and eating strategies that are exactly right for you. Here's to transforming your health, one easy step at a time.

Rachel Warren Chadd
Health Editor
Reader's Digest Books

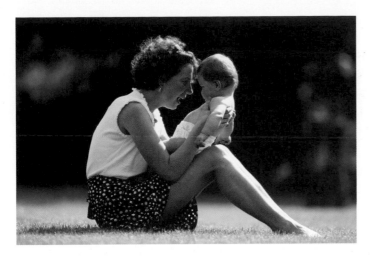

Better-than-ever health

Welcome to the first day of a new

beginning. You didn't ask for a

diabetes diagnosis, but it could

be the passport to a much healthier,

happier, energy-filled you.

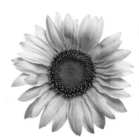

PLUS POINT Some people say diabetes helped them 'get their priorities right'.

The key to a healthier life

Most people with diabetes remember exactly when they were told they had it. It was likely to have been a defining moment filled with all sorts of emotions, including fear. Fear, of course, is a natural reaction to learning you have a chronic disease. It's what you do with that fear that makes the difference. You can let it defeat you, and put yourself at the mercy of whatever may come, or you can use it to fight back and reclaim your health. This book is about fighting back in small, easy ways every day – and reaping more rewards than you can possibly imagine.

Think of your Type 2 diabetes diagnosis as a wake-up call, a request from your body to take better care of your health. That doesn't mean you caused your diabetes; genes play a significant role. But it does mean you need to start eating more nutritious foods in reasonable-sized portions, being more active and even paying more attention to your stress levels and your nightly sleep habits. Diabetes isn't like a broken arm; you can't isolate the problem and let it heal while you carry on with life as normal. Controlling it means taking steps that affect your whole body. And when you take them, your body, mind and spirit will benefit.

In fact, some people with diabetes say they have become healthier than they were before they were diagnosed; that the disease helped them to 'get their priorities right'. They have better habits and happier lives, and they're more optimistic. They have greater energy and a stronger sense of personal control. You can, too, and it may take less effort than you think.

Have you noticed how giving a simple heartfelt compliment to your partner once in a while can cut down on arguments? That putting all your new bills in one place is the key to making sure they get paid? That having a store of birthday cards to hand removes all panic when you remember a birthday at the last minute? Equally small measures can help you to manage your diabetes better, and this book is packed with them. We'll take you through the tiny adjustments you can make in every part of your life – including areas such as your mind and your relationships. Just like that compliment, that dedicated bill drawer, and that store of birthday cards, they'll help you to head off problems, live better and cut down on unnecessary stress.

Let's be clear: it's your life to live and these are your habits to adopt. No health professional can adopt them for you. They can examine you, order blood tests, write prescriptions and talk to you during appointments about how you're doing. But the truth about any kind of healthcare is this: your health professionals cannot oversee the management of your diabetes day in and day out. And you wouldn't really want any of them in your kitchen (too many cooks), in your car (backseat driver), or at your desk at work (could they do your job?). Your team are advisers who can only suggest a plan of action. You're the one who will carry it out, from the time you wake up and start the day to the time you snuggle back into bed early enough to get a full night's sleep.

That doesn't mean you have to go it alone. In fact, you'll both want and need plenty of people in your corner, from health professionals (including your GP and diabetes specialist nurse) to your family and other people with diabetes. You'll read more about all of them later in the book.

But at the centre of this is one person: you. So seek every bit of help you can get in terms of professional guidance and support – then be prepared to take matters into your own hands. The sooner the better. The fact is, most people with Type 2 diabetes had it for several years before they were diagnosed. And Type 2 diabetes is a progressive disease; it tends to get worse over time. But with this book in hand, and more than 700 simple, clever tips at your disposal, you can get the better of it – and enjoy life like never before.

Diabetes: an exceptional disease

With most diseases, it's fairly easy to picture what's wrong and how to remedy it. If you have a broken arm, you put it in plaster. If you have an infection, you take antibiotics. Diabetes is different. The problems involved – at the core, an inability to produce and/or use enough of the hormone insulin to process the glucose, or blood glucose, that fuels your cells – are hard to visualise, which may make the disease seem less 'real'. But it's real all right. And the 'simple' problem of high blood glucose doesn't end with your blood. Diabetes has a cascade of effects, damaging a number of body systems as it progresses.

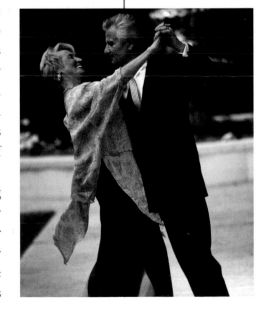

For the rest of your life, your diabetes is going to be somewhere along a spectrum: in the early stages, you may experience few symptoms or complications – you'll actually be relatively healthy. At the opposite end of the spectrum are the serious complications that result when this chronic disease goes unchecked – blindness, kidney disease, amputation, nerve damage, sexual dysfunction and heart disease, for instance. Among people with diabetes, 65 per cent die of heart disease or stroke. Diabetes causes 44 per cent of all cases of kidney failure, and 60 to 70 per cent of people with diabetes have some degree of nerve damage. Men who have diabetes are twice as likely to have erectile dysfunction as men who don't have diabetes.

Those figures are sobering indeed. But here's the silver lining: you can stop or slow your progress somewhere along the line at any time. You may even be able to reverse some of the damage. And it won't take a miracle – just simple determination and persistence.

Top habits to adopt

A diabetes diagnosis often brings with it a mind-numbing barrage of tablets, insulin and testing, meal plans and more. It's enough to set your blood pressure soaring, even if it was normal before. People can become frustrated by everything they have to do for their diabetes, and some get so overwhelmed that they feel paralysed and confused, so are unable to do anything well. 'Diabetes burnout' (frazzled to the point of giving up) is a major concern among health professionals.

Can you 'beat' diabetes?

We say you can. It's true that there's currently no cure for the disease. But you can reverse the core problems – insulin resistance and lack of insulin secretion – by tweaking what you eat and how often you exercise. If you can adjust your lifestyle, you could possibly even reduce your need for medication or insulin for a time.

You'll see results straightaway when you start following the advice in this book. In fact, you could see positive blood-glucose changes from some of the tips in a matter or days or even hours. Over time, making some of our strategies part of your daily routine could make the difference between, say, developing a foot ulcer or not.

Your efforts will have a profound effect. For instance, researchers say that for every one-point drop in your HbA1C blood glucose result (a measure of blood glucose over the last three months), you reduce your risk of eye, kidney and nerve damage by 40 per cent. Controlling your blood pressure when you have diabetes can reduce your risk of heart disease by as much as 50 per cent and of eye damage by 33 per cent. Also, simple and practical footcare to protect your feet from injury is known to significantly reduce the risk of amputation.

With results like that within your power, there's simply no reason why you'd want to sit back and do nothing.

In a way, this book is all about battling burnout. The tips are useful, easy and even fun, and there are many that you'll never have heard of before. You don't have to follow all of them, just choose a few to start with – maybe adding an extra vegetable serving at dinner and a short walk after your meal – then dip back into the book and add a few more when you're ready. They'll make a noticeable difference before you know it.

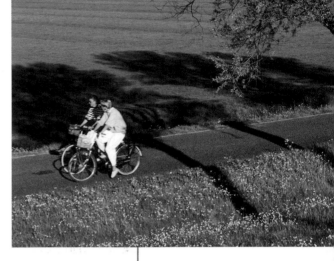

Many of our everyday tips are designed to help you do the things that matter most to your diabetes. For instance, many research studies show that losing just 10 per cent of your body weight (for instance, 8kg, or about 18lb if you weigh 80kg/12½st) – can reduce your insulin resistance, increase your insulin secretion and lower your blood glucose levels, essentially putting the disease in reverse. Here are some of the most important overall goals we'll help you accomplish. Of course, it's also absolutely critical to take the medicines you have been prescribed, on time and without fail.

Monitor your blood glucose

There's an old saying among people who study management: 'That which gets measured gets done.' Meaning, you are much more likely to achieve goals if you are getting constant feedback that plots the results of your efforts. In controlling diabetes, this means checking the glucose levels in a drop of your blood – possibly several times a day, depending on your situation. The results show you how your body is reacting to the foods you eat, the medications you take, how active you are and what level of stress you are experiencing. Manufacturers are bending over backwards to make testing as convenient and pain-free as possible, so stay alert to innovations in testing technology.

Keep calories under control

You will hear a lot of talk about sugar and carbohydrates as they pertain to diabetes, but the ultimate goal for most people is to reduce calorie consumption to a level that allows them to gradually lose weight if they need to. The most powerful way to do this and to get the nutrition your body needs is to eat plenty of fruit, vegetables and whole grains, while cutting back on red meat, ice cream, cakes and junk food. Of course, watching your portion sizes is also critical. Excess body fat is the most significant factor in the development of Type 2 diabetes, and losing weight is your first priority if you want to control the disease.

Eat the right carbohydrates

It's important to control the amount of carbohydrate you eat, because it's mainly carbohydrate foods that raise blood glucose, and you'll discover tips for finding and reaching your daily carbohydrate targets in this book. But changing the type of carbohydrates you eat might be just as important, as some carb foods raise blood glucose higher and faster than others. Eating foods that are lower on the glycaemic index – something you'll read about later on – has emerged as critical for keeping weight and blood glucose under control. It means switching to foods made from whole grains (such as wholemeal bread, porridge oats and wholemeal pasta) and cutting down on foods made from white flour (such as white bread, rolls and bagels) as well as other refined grains, such as white rice. It also means cutting down on foods made from grains that have been processed to the point where they're practically pre-digested (like brown breads that have the same look, feel and texture as white bread) and reducing the very starchy foods you eat, such as rice and potatoes, and drinking fewer sugary soft drinks, such as cola and lemonade.

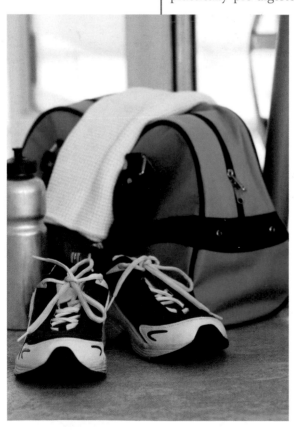

Get off the couch

We are in the midst of an epidemic of 'sitting disease'. Most of us move through a daily progression of sitting in the car, then sitting at our desks, then sitting in the car again, then sitting on the couch. All this sitting contributes to a bigger waistline, and obesity is one of the main factors fuelling the current explosion of diabetes in the developed world.

Being physically active is one of the most important things you can do for your body, your mind and your diabetes. When you move your body more, you burn more calories. You also build muscle, which boosts your metabolism. It's possible to lose weight through diet alone, but it's much easier when you combine calorie cutting with physical activity. Ideally, use a blend of aerobic exercise (walking, swimming, cycling and other heart-pumping activities) with strength training (weight lifting and calisthenics, for instance).

Exercise does more than help you to lose weight. Losing fat and increasing muscle makes cells more sensitive to insulin so they can take up more glucose and leave your blood glucose levels lower. That's why having a balanced diet and increasing physical activity are two of the most powerful tools in preventing or controlling Type 2 diabetes.

Aim to keep your blood glucose and blood pressure levels under control

Much of diabetes control focuses on keeping blood glucose as near as possible to the normal range. That's because this strategy has been shown to prevent damage to the eyes, kidneys and nerves – common complications of having diabetes. Other health problems often accompany high blood glucose, including high blood pressure, high cholesterol and high triglycerides, which all contribute to heart disease. In fact, high blood pressure can do more harm to your heart than high blood glucose.

Conveniently, the same strategies that help to control your blood glucose, such as moderate exercise, healthy eating and weight loss, will also do a world of good for the health of your heart.

Get support

If you've been reluctant in the past to have much to do with doctors and other health professionals, you'll have to adjust. You will need to build ongoing relationships with them so they can regularly evaluate aspects of your health, answer your questions and provide the tools and medications you need to control your diabetes. These professionals would typically include a doctor who specialises in diabetes, a diabetes specialist nurse or practice nurse, and a registered dietitian who will help you to establish a way of eating that's based on your goals and your tastes.

From time to time you will also need to consult an optometrist or eye specialist, a podiatrist and a pharmacist. In addition, a mental health professional can provide valuable advice for coping with the emotional issues that many people with diabetes face. Ensuring that you have the support of family and friends, and that you discuss the condition with other people who have diabetes will also help you to manage the condition successfully long term.

Keep the information flowing

Diabetes care is a true partnership between you and the diabetes health professionals and other staff with whom you come into contact. You are the centre of the team and the expert in your own life and your own diabetes. All the information that is held about you, and the decisions that are made about managing your diabetes need to involve you personally. Like the professionals, you also have a responsibility to collect, offer and receive information, and contribute equally in consultations, to help make the most relevant and useful decisions when you attend appointments.

Are you ready?

When you catch a cold, it will go away after a week or two. Having diabetes isn't like that. Unfortunately, your diabetes will never go away. It's there, even if you'd prefer to ignore it, and if you ignore it, it will get worse. On the other hand, if you accept the fact that diabetes is part of your life and decide to fight back, you can radically reduce your risk of diabetes-related health problems simply by adopting a few new habits here and there that will make you feel better – no matter what prompted you to try them. And when you feel good, you'll have the motivation and energy you need to implement a few more changes.

Before you know it, you could start to really appreciate the taste and texture of fresh whole foods; you could relish the 30 minutes in your day that you reserve for a mind-cleansing, stress-relieving walk; you could feel stronger; your clothes could fit better; and you could wake up in the morning with a more positive attitude. If you have to have diabetes, why not use it as an excuse to lead a healthier, more enjoyable life? This book offers you more than 700 ways to do it. Pick one and start today.

Rosie Walker RN BSc(Hons) MA(Ed)
Education Director
Successful Diabetes

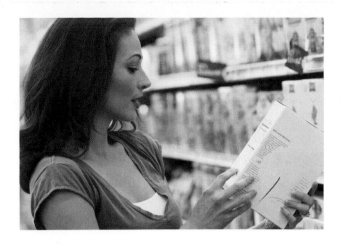

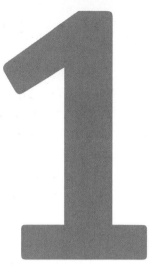

At the supermarket

When faced with the huge choice

available at the supermarket, it pays to

go armed with a plan. How you shop

influences how well you eat at home –

and even how well you manage

your diabetes.

Walk in with a plan

The most successful shopping trip starts before you even walk out of the door. That's because knowing what to buy means first knowing what you're going to eat. Your first job, then, is to do a bit of advance planning on the menu front. You'll also want to follow some of our 'smarter-shopping' tips to help you to plan a healthy diet.

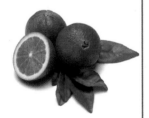

PLUS POINT

The better your diet, the better you will be able to control your blood glucose and possibly reduce your diabetes medications.

Shop with a detailed list in hand and cross off items as you shop. In the next chapter you'll read how important it is to plan your meals and you'll get some tips to help you do that. Make a shopping list based on the meals you've planned, and don't buy anything that isn't on the list, except for staples such as toilet paper and washing powder. With your list firmly in hand, you'll find no excuse to throw junk food into your trolley. Incidentally, studies show that people who plan their meals and make detailed shopping lists tend to eat more vegetables than those who don't.

Take a mental stroll around the shop before you put pen to paper. If you go to the same supermarket every week, you probably know the layout like the back of your hand. As you write your shopping list, think about the route you take around the aisles, and write your list out in that order. This way, you'll never have to backtrack through any department, helping you to avoid those impulse buys, such as the crisps you simply couldn't resist the third time you passed them.

Plan to spend most of your time in the fresh food sections of the supermarket. This is where you'll be able to pile up your trolley with fruit, vegetables and other fresh items. You'll need to visit other parts of the shop for olive oil, tinned tomatoes and pasta, but these items are not normally located in the same aisle as the processed foods that are so hard to resist. Simply steering clear of the crisp and biscuit aisles will do wonders for your willpower.

Do your nutritional sleuthing on the internet. The supermarket isn't a library – you don't have to spend your time at the store squinting at food labels. If you have a computer, you can do all the nutritional research you want to before you leave home. To help you make sense of food labelling, the British Nutrition Foundation has produced a basic guide, which is available on its website (www.nutrition.org.uk). Go to the Healthy Eating section and then to 'Food Science/Labels'. The Food Standards Agency also has a guide (www.foodstandardsagency.gov.uk), which you'll find under the section 'Labelling and packaging'. Most manufacturers list the nutritional information for all their products on their own websites. These are helpful tools if you are counting carbohydrates for blood glucose control. (For information about carbohydrate counting, see chapter 2.)

Eat a healthy snack before you leave the house. If your stomach is rumbling while you shop, you're more likely to come home with precisely what you shouldn't be eating – convenience foods in boxes and packages that are high in sugar, fat, or salt, or all three! But if you've just eaten a fresh summer peach before you get to the supermarket, it'll remind you to buy more of them while you're there.

Don't be afraid to pay more for fresh produce. You can be sure that your food bills will even out in the end because of the things you're not buying – namely, junk food. A 14-bag multi pack of crisps (25g per bag) can cost £2.26, which adds up to more than £6.50 per kilo – much more than a kilo of apples. A 500g bag of pearl barley is a give-away at 49p, while 500g of dried haricot beans for just 99p will last you for weeks, compared to an overpriced frozen ready meal that will be gone in a day. Remember that eating better now could help you to control your blood glucose better in the future.

Rate yourself when you get home. Look at your receipt and highlight your healthy food purchases: fresh and frozen fruits and vegetables, whole grains, low-fat dairy foods, dried or low-salt canned beans, lean meats, fish, nuts and olive oil. Most of your till receipt should be highlighted, with only a few lines of indulgent snacks and ready-made foods left out. Use this list as a starting point for an even healthier shop next week, either in the supermarket or online.

golden rule

Buy food your grandparents would have recognised

The chances are that at your age your grandparents would never have laid eyes on multicoloured fruit snacks, cereal bars coated in chocolate or frozen microwave pizza. But they certainly would have recognised fresh fruits and vegetables, meats and poultry, fish and other 'whole' foods in their natural state. So buy bananas instead of banana-flavoured pudding, pork chops rather than sausages, and fresh or bagged salad leaves rather than a ready-made Caesar salad with its own fat-laden dressing and croutons. Not only will you maximise your vitamin and mineral intake, you won't ingest the salt, sugar, harmful fats and chemical additives that are found in so many processed foods.

Linger in the fruit and veg department

It's no wonder that restaurants garnish their plates with parsley, tomato wedges and cleverly carved radishes – vegetables' vibrant colours add a bit of pizzazz to a meal. But what's more important is the nutritional benefit that vegetables offer: fibre, vitamins and disease-fighting antioxidants, and they're generally low in both calories and carbohydrates. If there's anywhere in the supermarket that you should allow yourself to make impulse purchases, it's here.

Designate a vegetable of the week. Tired of the same old tomatoes and carrots? Good! It's time to try something new, especially if a little variety helps you to eat more vegetables. To sneak in an extra serving of vegetables every day, buy a vegetable you've never tried – or one that you haven't eaten in a long time – then challenge yourself to work it into your diet every day that week. It could be as simple as broccoli or green beans or as exotic as bok choy. Your goal: have none of it left to throw away at the end of the week.

Take the free recipe. Many supermarkets give away recipes that spotlight fresh vegetables in an effort to get customers to eat (and buy) more of them. Usually the featured recipes are for seasonal, sometimes exotic vegetables. Take one and give it a try.

Darken your greens. It's smart to shake yourself out of the iceberg lettuce habit. Not only do baby spinach, rocket, watercress and green lettuces (Romaine, also known as Cos, and Little Gem) bring new crunch and flavour to your salads, they also add more vitamins. For example, a portion of iceberg lettuce contains 7 per cent of your daily vitamin A needs; a portion of raw spinach leaves is packed with more than 50 per cent, plus 14 per cent of your vitamin C needs.

golden rule

Fill up half your trolley with colourful produce

Colours indicate the presence of various phytochemicals, including antioxidants, which work together to neutralise free radicals, harmful molecules that your body may have in excess if you have diabetes. Free radicals wreak havoc on cells and can increase your chances of suffering diabetes-related complications and heart disease. The more intense the colour of the produce, the better. Choose bright red peppers and tomatoes, opt for orange with carrots, mangoes or cantaloupe, and go green with broccoli, kale and spinach. Your meals will also look and taste more interesting.

Splash out on pre-washed, pre-cut vegetables. A bag of ready-to-cook broccoli is more expensive than a fresh head of broccoli, and the same is true for pre-cut carrots, potatoes and peppers compared to those you have to peel, wash and slice yourself. But the investment can be well worth it if you're pressed for time, or if the preparation work puts you off eating vegetables at all.

Buy enough fruit and vegetables to last the week. That means three to five days' worth of fresh produce, supplemented with frozen or canned. 'I haven't shopped for a week' is no excuse for not getting at least five servings of fruit and vegetables per day. Frozen vegetables contain almost as many nutrients as their fresh counterparts – and they're easy to use. Adding a serving of frozen peas to your shepherd's pie, or two servings of frozen carrots to a curry, are simple ways to step up your vegetable intake.

Make your own vegetable ice cubes. These days you can even buy frozen onion but you may prefer to create your own frozen vegetables, preserving your home-grown or locally grown produce. Chop vegetables such as onions, celery, carrots, parsley or garlic, fill a plastic ice cube tray with them, add a little water (stock won't work), then freeze. Once they're frozen, put the cubes in a labelled plastic freezer bag or plastic box in the freezer. Add a cube or two to recipes as needed. This is also a good way to save produce that you can't use in time.

Mix and match your produce. Fruit and vegetables become more interesting when you eat them in unexpected combinations. Try shredded carrots with chopped mangoes, or pineapple with red onions, as toppings for grilled chicken breasts. Cauliflower and green grapes go together well to make a crunchy, tangy salad. Simply wash a head of cauliflower and break it into bit-sized florets. Toss it with four handfuls of halved green grapes and 50g toasted and coarsely chopped walnuts. Then add a dressing made by mixing 4 tablespoons fat-free or light mayonnaise, 2 tablespoons honey, and 1 tablespoon yellow mustard. You'll have enough for 10 servings.

whip it together!

Broccoli surprise salad

Broccoli and strawberries join together in this palate-pleasing salad packed with vitamins, fibre – and flavour.

In a bowl, mix together 150g fresh **broccoli florets**, 75g quartered **strawberries**, 2 tablespoons of sliced **almonds** or roasted **linseeds** (that's an extra 6g of fibre) and 25g shredded reduced-fat mature **cheddar cheese**. Prepare the dressing in a smaller bowl by mixing 2 tablespoons reduced-fat **mayonnaise**, ½ tablespoon of **sugar** or **sugar substitute** and 1 teaspoon **cider vinegar**. Pour over the salad and mix well.

Fill up on fruit

Bananas on your cereal. Strawberry smoothies. With treats as sweet as these, why do we find it so hard to eat more fruit? It's a gold mine for vitamins and minerals, especially vitamin C, which helps prevent the damage that high blood glucose does to cells and arteries.

Add more citrus fruit to your trolley. Oranges, lemons, limes and grapefruit aren't just rich in vitamin C, they're also surprisingly good sources of fibre. (One large orange contains 4g.) Lemon and lime juice are delicious in home-made salad dressings. The zest can be grated into vinaigrette dressings or added to the dry ingredients of breads and cakes. Preliminary research suggests that acidic foods such as lemon actually blunt the effect of meals on your blood glucose levels. Buy a few extra lemons and plan to add the juice to everything from tuna sandwiches to pasta dishes.

Bag some apples. Want to keep your blood glucose on an even keel? Heed the old saying about eating apples to keep the doctor away. Apples are loaded with soluble fibre, which slows the digestion of food and thus the entry of glucose into the bloodstream. One group of researchers discovered that women who ate at least one apple a day were 28 per cent less likely to develop diabetes than those who ate none. Apples are also rich in flavonoids, antioxidants that help to prevent heart disease – but you need to eat the skin, too.

Scoop up a cantaloupe. These melons are real stars in the vitamin C department. And despite their sweetness, melons do not contain a lot of sugar, so forget anything you've heard about banning them from your diet. Can't use up a whole cantaloupe by having a slice every morning with breakfast? No problem. Make up some sugar-free flavoured jelly crystals according to the packet's instructions, and add the leftover melon, cut into chunks. Leave to chill and you have an easy, low-fat dessert. A 100g portion of melon contains 16 per cent of your recommended daily allowance of vitamin A, essential protection against some of diabetes' major complications, such as kidney and retina problems.

Buy as many berries as you can eat in a week. Though sugary sweet in taste, their sweetness is deceptive. The natural sugar found in most fruits is fructose, which is sweeter than sucrose (table sugar), so it takes much less (with fewer calories) to get that sweet taste. And fructose is friendlier to blood glucose levels, causing a much slower rise than sucrose. Berries are packed full of fibre, too, not to mention anthocyanins, healthy plant compounds that scientists think may help to lower blood glucose by boosting insulin production.

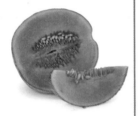

PLUS POINT

Cantaloupe is rich in vitamin A. It can protect you against some of diabetes' major complications.

Choose smarter carbohydrates

Carbohydrates aren't evil, despite their reputation. Yes, they do raise blood glucose levels, but cutting them out isn't the answer, for many good reasons. The trick is to control the types of carbohydrates you eat and how much of them you consume. You'll definitely want to up your intake of whole grains, not only for their fibre but also for their antioxidants, vitamins and minerals.

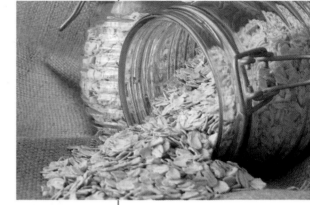

Choose cereal with at least 5g of fibre per serving. Among other benefits, fibre helps you to feel full so you can get through the morning with only a small snack, if anything, before lunch. Fibre from bran cereal is also associated with less inflammation in women with Type 2 diabetes. That is important because medical experts believe that inflammation plays a major role in diabetes as well as the development of heart disease. The US Physicians' Health Study found that doctors who ate whole-grain cereal every day over a period of 24 years were 28 per cent less likely to have heart failure.

Buy old-fashioned oats instead of instant cereals. If you're debating between porridge and a cold breakfast cereal such as cornflakes, choose porridge. It has fewer calories than most cereals, and is high in sugar-stabilising soluble fibre. In fact, research has found that eating a bowl of porridge five or six times a week can reduce the risk of getting Type 2 diabetes by 39 per cent. It also helps to lower cholesterol. But watch out for packets of instant porridge,

whip it together!

Pearl barley and chickpea salad

Don't shy away from buying pearl barley just because you don't know what to do with it. Try this delicious, fibre-rich salad, which is easy to put together from storecupboard staples.

Cook 120g **pearl barley** according to the packet's directions, then let it cool for about half an hour. In a bowl, combine the cooked barley with 1 can (410g) **chickpeas** (drained and rinsed), 10 sliced rehydrated **sun-dried tomatoes**, 1 tin (390g) **artichokes** (drained and halved), 3 finely chopped **spring onions** and 2 crushed **garlic** cloves. Mix well.

Toss with 100ml fat-free **Italian salad dressing**.

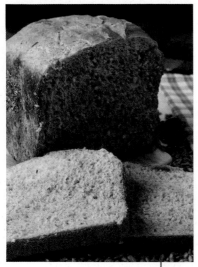

which usually contain added sugar, not to mention salt that can raise blood pressure. Flavoured instant porridge oats from a packet have up to 0.5g salt. A portion of porridge oats has only a trace of salt and you can always add your own flavours in the form of fruit (dried or fresh) and chopped nuts.

Choose bread with the word 'whole' in the first ingredient. Looking at the bread's colour won't tell you if it's really whole grain – you have to read the ingredient list. Look for bread made with wholemeal flour (stone ground is even better) or that has seeds or grains added. These breads will give you an extra fibre boost and also help to fill you up for longer. They also contain a higher amount of vitamins and minerals than other types of bread.

Enjoy chewy, dense loaves with visible kernels. Even if you choose a bread that's 100 per cent wholemeal, it may not be as friendly to your blood glucose as it could be. If the wheat has been finely ground to the point that the bread has the texture of white bread, it will be digested nearly as fast as white bread and will have similar effects on your blood glucose. Coarser grains take longer to digest and will raise blood glucose levels more slowly. Health-food shops will have this kind of bread if your local supermarket does not.

Look for extra-fibre breads. Some companies are selling bread with increased fibre and fewer carbohydrates: two slices contain the same amount of carbohydrates that are in one slice of regular bread. You can also find high-fibre bagels containing 8g of fibre per bagel. That's almost a third of your daily fibre target. Consuming 25g of fibre a day helps to lower cholesterol and control blood glucose.

golden rule

Aim to eat three servings of whole grains a day

Studies show that the more whole grains people eat, the greater their sensitivity to insulin and the lower their risk of developing diabetes. What's more, according to a study by medical researchers, consuming just two and a half servings of whole grains per day is associated with a 21 per cent lower risk of cardiovascular disease compared to consuming only 0.2 servings. What counts as a serving? One small slice of 100 per cent wholemeal bread, 40g porridge oats, or about 45g muesli.

Build up your stock of tinned beans and lentils. These are 'complex carbohydrates' that also supply protein without a lot of calories or fat, making them nearly perfect foods. Keep black beans, kidney beans, pinto beans, chickpeas, white beans and lentils on hand to add to your soups, salads and pasta dishes. Just tossing 200g of tinned chickpeas into tonight's salad will add an impressive 6g of fibre and 6g of protein.

Upgrade your pasta to whole wheat. You might think there's nothing worse for your blood glucose than pasta, but thanks to the durum wheat it's made from and the structure of the protein in pasta dough, that's not true. As it turns out, pasta has only a moderate effect on blood glucose levels – much more modest than that of the white Italian bread you might eat with your meal. But you'll get about three times the fibre per serving if you choose whole wheat. Not all brands and shapes taste as good in whole wheat; experiment to find one you like.

Eat brown rather than white rice. Like white bread, white rice is a refined carbohydrate, which will quickly convert to glucose in the body and send your blood glucose soaring. Brown rice, on the other hand, is a whole grain; 160g of cooked brown rice has 4g of fibre, compared to just 1g in white rice. Although even brown rice raises blood glucose more than porridge or barley, but it still offers the benefits of a whole-grain food.

Or buy basmati. This long-grained rice has a lower glycaemic index than other types of white rice, but it doesn't contain as much good-for-you fibre or as many nutrients as brown rice.

Buy some pearl barley. One of the most under-appreciated cereal grains, pearl barley can be used instead of rice or noodles in soups, stews and bean salads. Thanks to its impressive store of soluble fibre, which slows the digestion of food and therefore the rise of blood glucose, it's much friendlier to blood glucose than rice for most people. And it also lowers cholesterol levels.

whip it together!

Spinach and cannellini bean linguine

Make whole-wheat pasta interesting – and add fibre and nutrients – with this hearty, quick-to-fix dish. Canned salmon boosts the protein content and provides heart-healthy omega-3 fatty acids.

Bring a pan of water to the boil, **salt** lightly. Add 450g of **whole-wheat linguine** and cook for 7 minutes or until al dente. As it cooks, heat 1 tablespoon **olive oil** in a flat-bottomed pan. Sauté three minced **garlic** cloves in the oil for 30 seconds. Add 200g **baby spinach leaves** and sauté for 1 to 2 minutes. Stir in 1 tin (410g) **cannellini beans** (drained and rinsed) and 360g water-packed, reduced-salt, **canned flaked salmon**. Drain the pasta, reserving about 100ml of the cooking water. Add the cooking water to the spinach-garlic-bean mixture and mix. Add the sauce to the pasta and toss well. Season with **salt** and **pepper**.

Boost your dairy intake

Many of us haven't downed a glass of milk since we were children. We get our milk in dribs and drabs by adding it to coffee, cereal and tea. But eating more dairy foods is one of the most sensible things you can do to combat diabetes. Two recent studies found that people who made dairy foods part of their daily diets were 21 per cent less likely to develop insulin resistance and 9 per cent less likely to develop Type 2 diabetes. And research has found that the more calcium and vitamin D people get in their diets, the less likely they are to develop metabolic syndrome, which increases the risk of heart disease. Dairy foods may even help you to shed extra weight, which in turn helps your body to respond better to insulin and makes it easier for you to get your blood glucose under control.

Choose skimmed milk. Yes, whole milk tastes creamier, but one 200ml glass contains 9.5g of carbohydrate and 8g of fat (of which 5.2g are saturated). A 200ml glass of skimmed milk will give you all the calcium and vitamin D of the whole milk while saving you 66kcal and all the fat.

Wean yourself off fatty milk. You can start by buying milk that's one level down in fat. Switching straight from whole milk to skimmed in one step will be a big shock to your taste buds. Instead, first make the switch from whole milk to semi-skimmed milk. When your semi-skimmed milk is half gone, fill up the container with skimmed milk to make a milk type that's in-between the shop-bought ones. It will reduce the shock to your taste buds, when you finally move on to fully skimmed milk.

Buy some powdered skimmed milk. Stir a little into your glass of skimmed milk to give it more body and richness.

Keep a can of light evaporated milk to hand. It contains less than 1 per cent fat, so it's perfect for adding to coffee or using in recipes that call for cream. It even makes a tasty gravy: roast carrots, celery and onions

make the change

The habit: Getting at least four servings of calcium-rich foods a day.

The result: Potentially lowering your risk of developing metabolic syndrome, heart disease and other diabetes complications by about a third.

The evidence: US researchers studied the diets of 80,000 women in the Nurses' Health Study for more than 20 years and found that those who consumed more than 1,200mg of calcium and more than 20mcg of vitamin D a day had a 33 per cent lower risk of developing Type 2 diabetes compared with women who consumed less. In another study of more than 10,000 women aged 45 and older, getting more calcium and vitamin D lowered the risk of having metabolic syndrome, a cluster of symptoms that can lead to Type 2 diabetes and heart disease. Women with a higher calcium intake also had lower cholesterol. A 200ml glass of milk contains about 250mg of calcium – just choose the skimmed variety to curtail your intake of saturated fats.

and mash them. Then add a bit of flour to the pan and cook to make a roux. Put the mixture in a blender with a little evaporated light milk and reheat the mixture on the stove.

Use light evaporated milk to whip up a sweet topping. Instead of using whipped cream, pour in some light evaporated milk, then add a low-calorie sweetener to taste. Grab a whisk and whip away!

Choose fat-free, unsweetened (plain) yoghurt. Liven it up with your own healthy additions of fruit, nuts and seeds. This gives you the double benefit of avoiding the saturated fat in whole-milk yoghurt and the extra sugar in sweetened yoghurt. If you add, for example, 150g of fresh strawberries to plain yoghurt, you're adding 3g of fibre as well as plenty of natural fruit sweetness. For crunch, throw in some granola (found in the cereal aisle), muesli or ground linseeds.

Purchase low-fat cheese – selectively. Let's face it, some low-fat cheeses aren't worth eating. But if you're using cheddar in casseroles or on top of chilli, the low-fat versions will work just fine, and you won't really notice the difference. Using low-fat cheddar instead of regular will save you about 45kcal and 5g of saturated fat per 25g serving. This small switch goes a long way to cutting cholesterol and lowering your risk for heart disease.

Look sharp when it comes to cheese. Here's a secret that gourmet chefs use all the time: pick a strongly flavoured, pungent cheese such as extra-mature Cheddar or Parmesan and use only a little of it on top of pastas or salads. This trick will not sacrifice flavour, but it will save you money (the less you use, the more money you save) as well as artery-clogging saturated fat (since you'll be using less of it).

Put a carton of soya milk in your trolley. Soya milk, tofu and other soya products are good sources of calcium. In addition, soya protein has been shown to lower protein levels (a sign of better kidney function) in the urine of people with Type 2 diabetes while slightly improving levels of HDL or 'good' cholesterol. In one study involving overweight people who drank either dairy-based or soya-based meal replacement drinks, the soya group saw their blood glucose levels drop. Soya has also been shown to reduce the risk of some cancers. Avoid flavoured soya milks, though, which contain added sugar. Soya milk will last for about a week in the fridge after you open it.

Fill up with lean protein

Protein has little or no effect on your blood glucose, but you need to ensure you go for lean rather than fatty choices. Protein also helps to keep hunger at bay between meals, facilitating weight loss. That said, there's no need to go overboard and it is still important to ensure that you have a high-fibre carbohydrate source with each meal. Some doctors warn against consuming too much protein if you have diabetes because of the strain it puts on the kidneys (many people with diabetes are at high risk of kidney disease). And the saturated fat in red meat contributes to insulin resistance. The trick then, is to choose lean protein and, fortunately, that's a relatively easy task.

Head to the sushi section of the chiller cabinets for a protein-packed meal. If ever you need a quick, prepackaged meal, this is the place to stop. Sushi delivers protein and some fibre and is generally low in calories – one piece of California roll has just 30kcal and less than a 1g of fat. Just steer clear of the soy sauce, which is

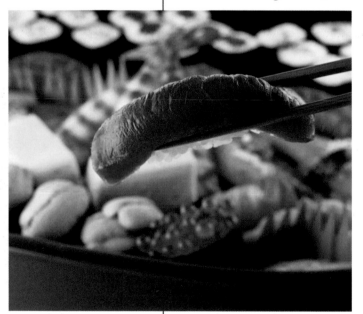

very high in salt, or ask for the low-salt variety.

Don't forget the eggs. Eggs have been much maligned over the years, but the fact is they are an excellent and inexpensive source of protein. One large, hard-boiled egg contains 7g of protein and has just 2g of saturated fat. To avoid the saturated fat altogether, use the egg whites and throw out the yolks. Or you can dress that egg up (and get in a serving of vegetables) by making an omelette and folding in spinach, which is rich in iron and fibre. In various studies, people who ate eggs and toast for breakfast stayed full longer and ate significantly fewer calories the rest of the day than people who ate, for example, a bagel and cream cheese. Eggs contain a fair amount of cholesterol, but dozens of studies have shown that it's saturated fat, not dietary cholesterol, that raises people's cholesterol the most.

Go for steak mince, it's often the leanest minced beef. But, be aware that there is a confusing array of definitions and 'lean' in one shop may be leaner than another. A recent Food Standards Agency survey tested the fat content of mince labelled as lean (which should have a 9 per cent fat content, unless otherwise stated) in several shops, and found shockingly that the actual fat content varied from 5 to 30 per cent. Many supermarkets now state the fat content of their prepackaged minced beef. If you buy your mince from a local butcher, ask for the leanest available.

Buy at most two servings of red meat per person per week. Red meat contains saturated fat, and one study found that women with Type 2 diabetes who ate more red meat were more likely to develop heart disease than women with diabetes who ate less. Other research showed that the more red meat women ate over a period of almost nine years, the more likely they were to develop Type 2 diabetes.

Avoid the bacon and sausages. While red meat seems to increase the risk of developing diabetes, processed meats such as bacon and sausages seem to increase it even more.

Pick up pork chops or pork tenderloin. Pork tenderloin is very lean meat and isn't too expensive. Put a couple of chops under the grill (dress them up with a low-calorie garlic-lime juice marinade, or with chilli and garlic powders) for a quick dinner – each is just 129kcal, with a healthy 16g of protein.

Beef – good and lean

On average, a lean cut of beef that has been fully trimmed contains less than 5 per cent fat. This is great news if you want to indulge in a steak or beef stew every now and again. It's important to balance your meal with some potatoes, pasta or rice and plenty of vegetables. The following cuts of beef are listed in order of leanness; a recommended serving is 100–150g (raw weight).

- Topside
- Stewing or braising steak
- Silverside
- Sirloin steak
- Rump steak
- Fillet steak
- Beef brisket
- Forerib of beef
- Beef flank

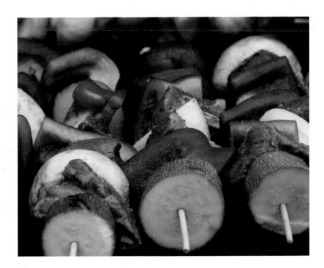

golden rule

Buy fresh fish every time you shop

Oily fish such as mackerel, sardines, herring, salmon and fresh tuna deliver plenty of protein without saturated fat – and they're excellent sources of omega-3 fatty acids, which help to cut the risk of heart disease. Equally important, they calm chronic inflammation, common in people with diabetes. (Several large studies found that women with the highest levels of chronic inflammation were four times as likely to develop Type 2 diabetes.)

Scientists aren't sure why, but inflammatory chemicals may interfere with the work of insulin, causing blood glucose to rise. So perhaps it's no coincidence that population studies show that fish lovers have unusually low rates of Type 2 diabetes. Your goal: eating at least two 85–140g servings of oily fish per week.

Buy a pack of chicken mini fillets to keep in your freezer. Each mini fillet weighs about 40-55g, which makes portion control easy: two mini fillets are roughly equal to one 85g serving, which is about the size of a pack of cards. The mini fillets will marinate quickly and can be used in kebabs or tossed into stir-fry dishes.

Choose turkey or chicken breast at the deli counter. Lean slices of meat on wholemeal bread topped with mustard and baby spinach leaves make a healthy, low-cholesterol lunch – that is, if you select lunch meats that are low in saturated fat. Avoid the salami and pepperoni. Good second choices are lean ham and roast beef – just stick to two slices or 40g of meat in your sandwich.

Go to the freezer section for frozen soya beans. These young green soya beans, in or out of their shell, are wonderful as snacks; just steam or boil them and add a little salt. You can also add them to soups, sauces and salads. Soya has more protein, by volume, than beef, and virtually none of the saturated fat.

Buy canned fish, too. Salmon is nature's heart medicine, but you don't have to cook up a fillet to get more of it into your diet. Tinned salmon is a smart choice not only for convenience but for health; make sure any tinned salmon is wild and not farmed as it contains fewer contaminants. An added incentive for eating salmon that researchers found was that people who had the highest levels of omega-3 fatty acids in their blood were 53 per cent less likely to report feeling mildly or moderately depressed.

Buy seafood to store in the freezer. Vacuum-packed fish that have been flash-frozen at sea are the next best thing to fresh fish.

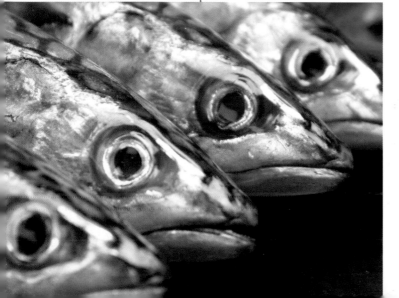

However, be careful to check that the fish has been sustainably caught and is not on an endangered list. The packaging should have the 'Marine Stewardship Council' logo on it. A full list of endangered fish can be found at www.fishonline.org. Packs of cleaned frozen prawns are another great buy. Mix prawns with frozen mixed vegetables and you have the makings of a stir-fry dinner ready to go.

Shop for healthier snacks and sweets

Snacking isn't right for everyone who has diabetes, but for some people, especially those who go more than four or five hours between meals, and take insulin or insulin-stimulating tablets, snacks have a place on the menu. The trick is to choose healthy munchies. Unfortunately, many of the items in the 'snack aisle' are filled with cheap ingredients such as high-fructose corn syrup and hydrogenated oil that do little or nothing for you except increase your consumption of empty calories, dangerous fats and refined carbohydrates, which wreak havoc on blood glucose and contribute to weight gain. Here's how to select treats that indulge your sweet and salty cravings but won't lead you to put on weight or raise your blood glucose levels.

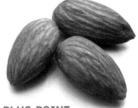

PLUS POINT
Even though nuts are high in calories, people who eat them tend to weigh less.

Head back to the fruit and vegetable section. This is where you'll find pre-sliced, pre-washed carrot sticks. It's even better (and cheaper) to make your own. Pop them in the front of your fridge or take them with you in a zip-lock bag when you're on the go for a healthy snack anywhere, anytime. With all their fibre and water, carrots fill your tummy with very few calories.

Say yes to low-fat mini cheeses. Snacks low in carbohydrates and moderate in fat are rare, but this is one of them. Though the mini cheeses may be more expensive gram for gram than buying a block of cheese, they are a sound nutritional investment. The 21g servings contain just 50kcal, 4g of fat and no carbohydrate. You'll know exactly how much cheese you're eating rather than guessing the amount you have taken from a large block.

Buy single-serving boxes of raisins. Yes, raisins are higher in sugar than the grapes from which they come. But single-serving boxes will make sure that you stick to small portions of this otherwise good-for-you food.

Go nuts (in moderation). Even though nuts are high in calories, studies show that people who eat nuts tend to weigh less. And Harvard researchers found that women who regularly ate about a handful of nuts five times a week were 20 per cent less likely to develop Type 2 diabetes than those who didn't. The benefits probably come from the blend of protein and good-for-you fats that nuts contain, which make them an ideal snack. Just be sure to buy the no-salt versions. Almonds in particular are excellent sources of vitamin E, an antioxidant that may protect against kidney damage, and also against eye and nerve complications.

Choose low-fat, whole-grain crackers. If the cracker you usually eat leaves a ring of oil when you set it down on a napkin, then you know it's time to change. Buy a brand that contains at least 3g of fibre per serving (about six small crackers). Make sure it doesn't contain any trans fats (check for the word 'hydrogenated' on the ingredient list), which have been linked to heart disease.

Choose cereal bars carefully. Some cereal bars, with lots of added sugar and little fibre, might as well be chocolate bars. But if you look hard, you can find a brand that contains no less than 6g of fibre and no more than 100kcal per bar. Some high-fibre bars contain as many as 9g of appetite-curbing fibre. It also doesn't hurt to see what effect your favourite cereal bar has on your blood glucose; try to check your blood glucose 2 hours after eating one. Once you find a good brand, buy a box and keep a few in your handbag or in your glove compartment for quick on-the-go snacks.

Ignore offers on unhealthy snacks. A 'buy one, get one free' offer on crisps may sound too good to miss, but it isn't. If you take them home (even if you have the intention of buying them for someone else in the house), you're bound to eat them.

Ignore the fat-free biscuits. Manufacturers usually just add more sugar to these, and research shows that most people will eat more of them than they would normal biscuits.

golden rule

Check food labels for saturated fat and salt

For people with diabetes, these are the crucially important pieces of data. Why? Diabetes puts you at a higher risk of developing heart disease so no more than 7 per cent of your calorie intake should come from saturated fat (for a 2,000kcal-a-day diet, that's a maximum of 15g of fat). And because having diabetes typically means having higher blood pressure, your intake of salt should not exceed 6g per day. Some labels will list grams of sodium. To convert this to salt, multiply the figure by 2.5.

Resist 'sugar-free' ice cream. Manufacturers sometimes use sugar alcohols as sweetening agents in sugar-free products, which can cause wind and diarrhoea. People with diabetes may already have decreased efficiency in their intestines; these foods could make their digestive troubles worse. In addition, sugar alcohols contain calories, and they can raise blood glucose. Enjoy a small portion of a reduced-fat ice cream or frozen yoghurt instead.

Get your chocolate fix from frozen chocolate milk sticks. These are only 71kcal per stick with 1.5g of fat and a much better bet than chocolate bars if you are watching your waistline.

Snack on dark chocolate chips. To satisfy a chocolate craving, eat five or six of the semi-sweet chips used to make chocolate-chip cookies. Dark chocolate is rich in antioxidants that protect your heart as well as the rest of your body from cell-damaging free radicals.

Sugar by any other name

Sugar is a simple carbohydrate devoid of any nutritional benefits. And even if an ingredient label doesn't list 'sugar' that doesn't mean there isn't any in the product. Manufacturers use more kinds of sugar than you can shake a stick at, and it's worth familiarising yourself with some of them so you're not fooled into thinking a food is better for you than it is. Look for any of these

- ● Sucrose
- ● Glucose
- ● Fructose
- ● Maltose
- ● Hydrolysed starch
- ● Invert sugar
- ● Corn syrup
- ● Honey

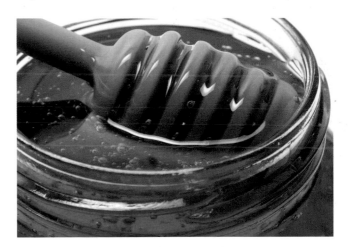

To get a sense of how much sugar you're really eating, check the nutrition label for 'sugars,' listed in grams. Every 4g is equivalent to a teaspoon of sugar. Experts suggest we limit our sugar intake to just 12 teaspoons a day from all food sources.

Shopping for low GI foods

What's the difference between mashed potatoes and spaghetti? The potatoes tend to send blood glucose up high in a hurry, while the pasta causes less of a rise – even if you were to eat the same amount of total carbohydrate in both cases. Scientists have discovered that some types of carbohydrates, once in the body, convert faster to glucose than others do.

Back in 1981 a nutrition scientist tested a group of people with a host of foods (all containing 50g of carbohydrate), measured their blood glucose reactions, and used them to rate the foods on a scale he called the glycaemic

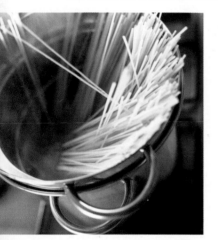

index (GI). He discovered that certain starchy foods, such as potatoes and cornflakes, raised blood glucose nearly as much as pure glucose did. These earned high GI scores.

One thing the GI doesn't take into account, is how much carbohydrate a serving of a food contains. You'd have to eat a lot of carrots to get 50g of carbs. The same goes for most vegetables and fruits. A better measure, then, is the glycaemic load (GL), which corrects for this problem.

Why are low-GL foods more desirable than high-GL foods?

High-GL foods cause blood glucose levels to rise sharply, prompting the pancreas to secrete insulin to bring it back down. Low-GL foods create a smaller, more sustained rise in blood glucose and don't require as much insulin. Studies have found that people whose diets have a high GL have a higher rate of obesity, diabetes, heart disease and cancer. One study found that men who typically ate high-GL foods had a 40 per cent higher chance of developing diabetes. In the Nurses' Health Study, women who ate diets with a high GL had a 37 per cent higher chance of getting Type 2 diabetes over the six-year span of the study. Yet another study found that exchanging just one baked potato per week for a serving of brown rice could reduce a person's odds of developing Type 2 diabetes by up to 30 per cent.

Of course, eating low-GL foods can also help if you already have diabetes. In one recent study published in the *American Journal of Clinical Nutrition*, researchers asked volunteers to eat 14 different typical meals (popular US fare, such as bagels and cream cheese with orange juice), then measured the change in their blood glucose levels. They found that the GI of the foods in each meal was about 90 per cent accurate in predicting how much the volunteers' glucose levels changed.

Can I lose weight eating lower-GL foods?

You may be able to. Because low-GL foods don't trigger blood glucose highs – which are usually followed by lows that cause hunger –

low-GL foods keep people feeling full longer. Population studies have shown that those who get most of their carbohydrates from the low end of the GI index tend to weigh less than others who gravitate towards high-GI sugary or starchy foods.

One study that compared a low-fat diet with a low-GL diet found that over the course of six to ten weeks, the people on the low-GL diet reported less hunger, showed better use of insulin, and had less inflammation in their bodies, which are all positive findings that translate into a lower risk of artery damage and heart disease.

How do I choose low-GL foods?

First and foremost, choosing low-GL foods means reaching for more fresh, non-starchy fruits and vegetables, nearly all of which fall very low on the GL scale. (Go easy on starchier vegetables including potatoes, parsnips, sweetcorn and peas.) Low-fat dairy foods also tend to be low-GL, along with most protein foods (that makes sense, as it is carbohydrates, not proteins, that raise blood glucose). Choose breakfast cereals with at least 5g of fibre per serving, and they are likely to be fairly low GL.

And make sure that you choose whole grains (such as brown rice, barley, bulghur, oats and coarse wholemeal bread) rather than refined grains such as white rice and white bread and foods made with white flour, such as most store-bought baked goods. In general, the more finely ground the grain and the less fibre it contains, the faster it will be digested – and the faster blood glucose will rise. That's one reason porridge, which isn't ground, has a lower GL than most breakfast cereals.

Which high-GL foods should I avoid?

Nutritionists say 'never say never'. In other words, no foods are banned completely from a healthy diet. See the chart below for a few foods to cut back on or eat in smaller portions and some comparable choices that don't raise blood glucose as much.

Instead of ...	Try
White potatoes or chips	Sweet potatoes or wedges made from sweet potatoes
White rice	Brown or basmati rice, quinoa, bulgur, pearl barley, or pasta cooked al dente
White bread	Coarse whole-grain bread, genuine sourdough bread, or dense rye bread
Cornflakes, rice cereal	Bran cereal or porridge
Sweetcorn	Beans and lentils
Crisps, pretzels, rice cakes or jelly beans	Nuts
Sugary drinks or fruit juices	Skimmed milk or tomato juice

For more information on the GL of common foods, see page 262.

Herbs, spices and extras

It's often the little things we add to our food that transform a meal from humdrum to high flavour. Herbs and spices are especially valuable, not only because they add taste without fat but also because many have strong antioxidant and anti-inflammatory powers.

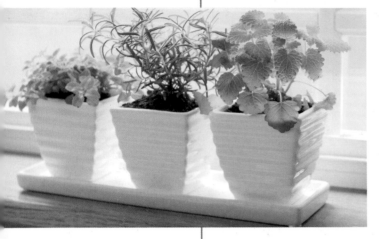

Condiments, such as mayonnaise and mustard, add tang and texture, but be careful in the condiment aisle or you could end up eating a lot more sugar and salt than you realise.

Buy potted herbs for your kitchen windowsill. If your local supermarket sells fresh flowers, it probably also sells potted plants – including culinary herbs. Herbs such as oregano, basil, thyme and rosemary will not only make your kitchen smell nice, they'll also be within easy reach when you want to flavour your meats and soups.

Build up your herb and spice supply with a new selection every week. Do you like your foods hot and spicy or herby? Whatever the case, adding variety to your spice rack can help you to add flavour to your food without calories or fat. The next time you're out shopping, bring home ginger, cayenne, turmeric, fresh garlic, curry leaves, dried basil, oregano and rosemary – or something completely new – and look for clever ways to work them into your meals. For instance, stir half a teaspoon of ground cumin into water before you boil some brown rice, add a little ginger to a hot lemon drink or sprinkle a little cinnamon over your porridge.

Look out for fruit and vegetable-based salsas. A Mexican favourite, salsa is a wonderful low-calorie, versatile condiment which instantly supplies a tasty topping for baked fish, chicken fajitas and baked potatoes. One 2 tablespoon serving from a jar of tomato-based salsa contains 10kcal and no fat. Think about that the next time that you reach for the mayonnaise – 2 tablespoons contain 114kcal and 10g of fat.

Seek out linseeds. You can easily add more fibre to any meal or snack by adding 1 or 2 teaspoons of ground linseeds. An easy way to remember their benefits is '1-1-1': each teaspoon of linseed has 1g of fat, 1g of fibre and 1g of protein (and only 17kcal). Purchase ground seeds or grind your own in a clean coffee grinder. Add them to smoothies, salads, casseroles and baked goods. Just make sure you store them in the refrigerator after opening. A word of warning: eat too many linseeds and you'll quickly discover their laxative effect.

Read condiment labels for calories and salt. If a tablespoon of the condiment contains less than 25kcal, you probably don't need to bother counting those carbohydrates (see page 52). But with some condiments, such as mayonnaise or mustards mixed with oils, the calories can add up fast, so buy something else, or plan to use it in very small portions. Salt is the other hidden hazard. A tablespoon of ketchup can contain around 0.5g of salt. Some salad dressings are even bigger offenders. Choose low-salt (or low-sodium) versions whenever possible (or make your own salad dressing).

Choose mustard over ketchup. Most mustards contain no added sugar, and they're much lower in salt than ketchup is.

Substitute low-fat yoghurt for mayonnaise. Save yourself some calories and help your waistline by mixing a small pot of natural yoghurt with the juice of half a lemon and some chopped basil, which makes a great alternative to mayonnaise in sandwiches. It can also be used as a tasty dip.

Grab a few heads of garlic. It appears to be a particularly beneficial herb for people with diabetes. Scientific studies show that garlic may increase insulin secretion, which lowers blood glucose; garlic also modestly lowers 'bad' cholesterol and 'thins' the blood to help prevent dangerous clots. And it's packed with antioxidants, which help to stave off diabetes-related complications. With its flavour and health benefits, garlic should be one of the first items you toss into your shopping trolley. It's delicious roasted and used as a spread on meat or bread. Minced garlic, too, jazzes up salad dressings, sautéed vegetables, meat marinades and more.

Stock up on lemon pepper. It's a wonderful way to add flavour, not salt, to vegetables, meats and starches.

Switch to rock salt. Because it's coarser, there's less of it by volume compared to normal table salt. In fact, there's nearly half the sodium in 1 tablespoon of rock salt than in table salt.

Try Cajun seasonings. These spice mixes lend serious kick without fat or calories to fish, chicken or prawns. They usually contain cayenne pepper, black pepper, garlic and onion powder, and possibly paprika, celery or fennel seeds, and other ingredients. If you like spicy food that's not too hot, there's no better way to add a lot of flavour. Also try other dry rubs, such as cracked pepper rubs. Go for the better brands; they often rely less on salt for their taste.

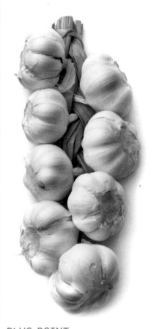

PLUS POINT
Garlic may increase insulin secretion, which lowers blood glucose.

Navigate the drinks aisle

If you have diabetes, working out what to drink can be tricky. Soft drinks (other than diet varieties) contain far too much sugar and too many calories, and even 100 per cent fruit juice should be rationed because it's higher in sugar than real fruit and contains none of the fibre. Read on for some suggestions.

Buy pomegranate juice and dilute it. This juice is especially high in antioxidants, but like other fruit juices, it's too high in calories. Dilute it with water (at least 50 per cent) and ice.

Stock up on tea. If you're limiting your intake of cola and other fizzy drinks, and you don't always care for plain water, what can you drink? Tea. It's rich in antioxidants that help to protect your arteries and stave off complications of diabetes. For a refreshing drink on a hot summer's day, make up some tea, let it cool, then add ice, lemon juice and a slice of lemon. You can, of course, also buy bottled and canned unsweetened iced teas but try to avoid the sweetened varieties.

Buy cordial (squash). Sugar-free cordial is one of the best and cheapest ways of making yourself a long, cool drink. If you make water taste good, you'll be likely to drink more of it.

Try tomato juice. It's a good way to sneak a vegetable serving into your day, and it has less of an effect on blood glucose than fruit juices do. That said, tomato juice tends to be high in salt, so look for a low-salt variety or add water to dilute it.

If you buy soft drinks, make sure they're diet ones. Fizzy drinks are filled with calories but empty on nutrition. Drinking them raises the risk of both diabetes and obesity. If you drink fizzy pop, make sure it is a diet variety and spare yourself the calories.

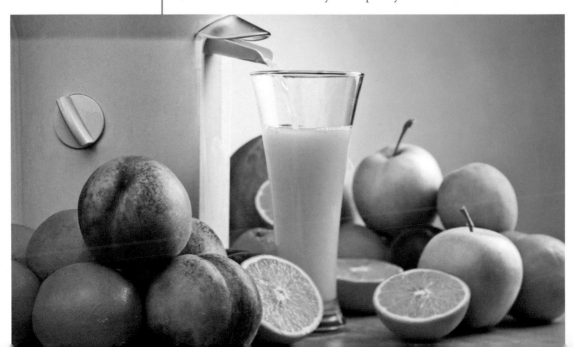

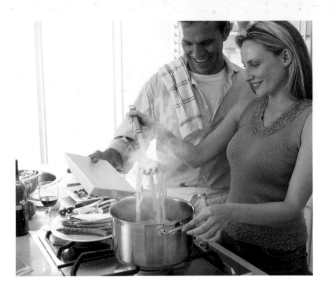

2

In your kitchen

Think of your kitchen as the control

room for managing your diabetes.

After all, in many ways this is a disease

that is closely linked with food. In this

chapter you'll learn the top strategies

for master-minding a culinary

campaign to beat diabetes.

Stock and streamline your cooking space

If success at any goal starts with a responsive mind, success at beating diabetes begins with a responsive kitchen. It's a simple law of human nature: the easier and more convenient it is to do something, the more likely you are to do it. Your aim is to set up a kitchen that lets you whip up healthy meals in a hurry, and keep healthy snacks and drinks readily to hand. Here's how to plan a kitchen that meets all your needs.

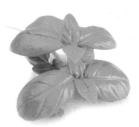

PLUS POINT
Many herbs and spices have powers that can help you to control diabetes.

Keep the kitchen clean. Make a rule and impress it on all family members: dirty dishes are never to be left in the sink, and the worktops and table must remain clean. You'll be far more motivated to cook healthy meals if you don't have to clean the kitchen first.

Place an enticing jug of water in the fridge. Look out your prettiest jug, fill it with ice, water and lemon wedges, and place it in your fridge in full view. Whenever you open the refrigerator out of boredom, pour yourself a glass of water. Researchers in Germany studied people's metabolism after they drank about 500ml of water. Within 10 minutes of taking the drink, they burned 30 per cent more calories than before they drank the water, and the boost in their metabolism lasted for 30 to 40 minutes. Another bonus is that water flushes impurities from your body, which is important for people with diabetes, who have a high risk of developing kidney disease. Drinking plenty of fluids also protects against water retention, a common problem when kidneys aren't functioning at their best.

Keep a bowl of fruit on the worktop. Make sure that fruits such as apples, pears, peaches and kiwis are the first foods you see when you enter the house ravenous at the end of the day or pop into the kitchen for a snack. A shallow bowl is better than a deep one because most fruits keep best unstacked. But in hot weather limit the amount of fruit kept out of the fridge as it will go off more quickly.

Stock the spice rack. Spices will help you to flavour your meals without adding fat or calories. Keep dry rubs for meats, Italian seasoning and other favourites in a spice rack on your kitchen worktop or tucked in your cupboard door for easy access. Some spices, including ginger, cayenne, turmeric, fresh garlic, curry powder, basil, oregano and rosemary, have anti-inflammatory and antioxidant powers, which help with diabetes. Keep them handy to flavour meat and vegetables.

Save a special place for cinnamon sticks. Some US doctors now believe that cinnamon should be the one spice that you reach for every day. Recent research has suggested that cinnamon may improve blood glucose levels and blood fats in people with Type 2 diabetes. More research is required and it is not advisable to take large doses of the spice, although using a little cinnamon regularly in your cooking may prove beneficial. And it will undoubtedly impart a wonderful flavour to your food.

Keep a small bottle of olive oil within easy reach. Olive oil is rich in healthy monounsaturated fats, which, unlike the saturated fat in butter, won't increase your insulin resistance (which raises blood glucose) and will protect your heart from heart disease. Because heat and light can turn olive oil rancid over time, keep a larger bottle in the fridge to refill your worktop bottle. Olive oil becomes cloudy in the fridge, but bringing it to room temperature will restore its clarity. Use extra-virgin olive oil. Because extra-virgin olive oil comes from the first pressing of olives and contains no refined oils, it has high levels of phenols – antioxidants that help prevent high cholesterol, high blood pressure and heart disease, as well as complications of diabetes, such as nerve problems.

Use a margarine that's free of trans fats. Trans fats, which are made when vegetable oils are hydrogenated and turned into solid fats, are considered deadly by many experts because they significantly increase the risk of heart disease. If you have high cholesterol, opt instead for a spread that contains plant sterols or stanols – they can actually block the amount of cholesterol absorbed by the gut.

make the change

The habit: Switching to olive oil.

The result: Lower blood pressure and cholesterol.

The evidence: In a study of men who don't normally consume olive oil, adding about 2 tablespoons a day to their diets over three weeks lowered their systolic blood pressure (the first number in a blood pressure reading) by 3 per cent. This is especially important for people with Type 2 diabetes because the disease puts you at higher risk of developing high blood pressure. In a separate study, adding 2 tablespoons of olive oil a day for six weeks led to a 12 per cent drop in total cholesterol and a 16 per cent drop in LDL ('bad' cholesterol). Olive oil also raises HDL, or 'good' cholesterol. Another healthy option is canola (or rapeseed) oil, also rich in mono-unsaturated fat and usually cheaper. Remember that 2 tablespoons of oil contain approximately 270kcal, so you'll need to use the oil in place of, not in addition to, other fats.

Throw away your corn oil. Corn oil doesn't compare well to olive oil when you examine their health benefits. Olive oil contains 72 per cent monounsaturated fats, while corn oil contains only 24 per cent, so olive oil does a better job of lowering cholesterol. Even more important, olive oil fights inflammation in the body, which is linked to many diseases including diabetes and heart disease, whereas corn oil is thought by many health experts to promote inflammation. When olive oil won't work in a recipe, such as in baking, use canola (also known as rapeseed) oil. It has a milder taste than olive oil but also contains an impressive amount of heart-healthy monounsaturated fat.

Keep several kinds of vinegar on hand. Cider, white, rice, balsamic and red and white wine vinegars will come in handy for

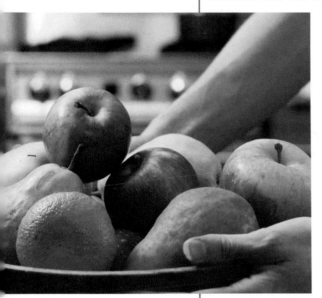

making quick salad dressings and marinades for meat or vegetables. And they bring an extra bonus: some early research suggests that adding acids to meals (such as vinegar or lemon juice) blunts the effect of the meal on your blood glucose. Try balsamic vinegar on top of sliced strawberries for an unexpected taste sensation.

Place healthy snacks within sight. You know you shouldn't be eating biscuits, so why did you pop one into your mouth the second you walked into the kitchen? Maybe because the open packet was sitting in the front of your cupboard, taunting you. Banish the biscuits to the back of a high shelf or even the freezer. Put in their place some almonds, walnuts and peanuts. Also keep some low-fat yoghurt in the front of the fridge, and store some cut-up carrot sticks or a bowl of cherry tomatoes or sugarsnap peas there, too.

Better yet, banish junk food from the kitchen. If your family insists on having bags of sugary, salty, fatty snacks around the house, ask them to keep the snacks where you won't find them. Hiding places outside the kitchen are best. Ask your partner to put his or her crisps in the garage or even locked in the boot of the car.

Stock some meal replacement drinks. You'll read on page 44 how important it is to eat breakfast every day. 'Real' food is always preferable to meal replacement drinks, but for those mornings when you don't have time even for a bowl of cereal, it's worth keeping some canned drinks or shakes ready to grab and go. Meal replacements such as SlimFast or a fruit smoothie are good alternatives. They usually contain protein and complex carbohydrates, and often some fibre as well, so they don't cause blood glucose to rise quite as high or as fast as other similar drinks.

Keep at least one emergency meal in the freezer. Forgot to buy chicken for Tuesday night's chicken marsala? No sweat. Individual servings of vegetable lasagna await in the freezer. Just heat and serve. When you run out of back-ups, make a double batch of your next meal and freeze the extra. Casseroles, soups and cooked meat can be frozen for up to three months. Use plastic bags and wrap made for the freezer or keep in airtight freezer containers.

Buy a vegetable steamer. Steaming is the healthiest way to cook vegetables because important nutrients aren't lost in the water. Choose a metal steamer basket (then fill it with vegetables, place over a saucepan of rapidly simmering water, cover, and cook for 5 to 10 minutes) or a microwave steamer (add a small amount of water to the bottom of the container, add vegetables to the basket, and cook for two to five minutes).

Keep an electric spice or coffee grinder on the worktop. Any of them will grind whole linseeds and make it convenient for you to add these important sources of fibre and omega-3 fatty acids to your cereal, salad, yoghurt and baked goods. Although you can buy ground linseeds, they won't be as fresh or tasty.

whip it together!

Cook-and-freeze turkey rice casserole

One bowl, one oven and one freezer. Could cooking be any simpler? Prepare this fibre-rich casserole when you have some extra time. On days when you can't spare a minute to cook, pop it out of the freezer and into the oven.

300g cooked **brown rice**

1 can (340g) **sweetcorn**, drained

250g diced **turkey breast**

1 **onion,** peeled and chopped

110g grated **reduced-fat Cheddar cheese**

240ml **skimmed milk**

½ teaspoon **chilli powder**

Salt and **pepper** to taste

Combine all ingredients in a large bowl. Pour into a nonstick 2 litre casserole dish. Bake at 180°C for 40 to 45 minutes. Remove from the oven, allow to cool slightly, cover and wrap in clingfilm. Place in the freezer for up to 2 months. When ready to serve, place in the fridge and thaw overnight. Bake at 160°C for 25 minutes until heated through.

Plan your meals

You wouldn't start a holiday without any idea of where you're going to go, and neither should you start your day or week without a clear idea of what you're going to eat. We're not saying you have to plan every bite, but with so many unhealthy choices all too readily available (you probably pass fast-food outlets whenever you drive your car and stare at chocolate bars when you buy your morning paper), having a plan, writing it down and sticking to it is a good approach.

Set aside time on Sunday to plan your menu for the next seven days. Look through cookbooks, recipe cards, websites or the latest issue of a healthy cooking magazine, and pick out seven healthy dinners with reasonable calorie totals, usually no more than about 500kcal per serving. Remember to include a lean protein source (such as chicken breast, fish or beans), plenty of vegetables, and a whole-grain source of fibre. Breakfasts and lunches can be a little more spontaneous, but it's still good to have a general idea of what you'll be eating (porridge or cereal with fruit in the mornings, salads and soups for lunch, etc) so you're never caught off guard and unprepared.

Write out a shopping list based on your week's menu. Take it to the supermarket and don't buy anything that's not on the list (unless, of course, you forgot to write down basics, such as milk and toilet paper). Now, even if your week turns busy and exhausting, you won't have to shop or wonder what you should make for dinner. A healthy meal is already planned and ready to cook.

Buy a set of magnetic clips and use them to hang your recipes for the week on the fridge. It will be one more reminder that you have a healthy meal planned before you have a chance to open the drawer in search of a take-away menu.

Put fish on the menu twice a week. Eating up to two servings of fish – especially oily fish such as salmon, tuna or mackerel – will supply enough omega-3 fatty acids to cut your risk of dying of a heart attack by 30 per cent. One way omega-3 fatty acids help to lower heart attack risk is by fighting inflammation in the arteries and elsewhere. Another advantage of 'fin food': if you're eating fish, that means you're not eating a fatty steak or an oversized plate of macaroni cheese, which is a diabetes disaster.

Enjoy a Greek 'picnic' on Thursdays. Start with a home-made Greek salad that includes lettuce, chopped juicy tomatoes, cubed cucumbers, a handful of chickpeas, 75g of grilled chicken per person and 25g of low-fat feta cheese per person. Drizzle with olive oil and vinegar and add a few sweet piquant peppers (sold in jars), if you like

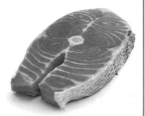

PLUS POINT
Eating oily fish can cut your risk of dying of a heart attack.

Secrets from a chef with diabetes

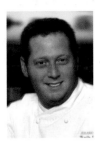

What does a chef do when he learns he has diabetes? Franklin Becker, chef of the Brasserie restaurant in New York City and author of *The Diabetic Chef*, put his cooking skills to the test. A lover of double plates of pasta and multiple slices of pizza, Becker decided to overhaul his eating habits, adding serious amounts of vegetables and cutting back on carbohydrates. Soon his body began adapting. He felt fuller on smaller portions, and he felt more energised.

Today, he has good control over his blood glucose levels. Here are a few of his tried and trusted recipes.

Downsized pizza Brush a flour tortilla with olive oil and layer with thin slices of tomatoes, grated low-fat mozzarella cheese and fresh basil. Heat in the oven until the cheese melts.

Steamy, tasty vegetables Add a bit of water to a saucepan with a teaspoon of olive oil, sea salt and any kind of vegetable, such as sugarsnap peas, broccoli or cauliflower. Cook the water and oil down until it thickens and forms a bit of a sauce. Finish it off with chopped fresh parsley, chives and tarragon.

Orange and rocket salad Toss rocket leaves with orange segments, freshly squeezed lemon and a drizzle of olive oil. 'The lemon cuts through the peppery taste of the rocket, and it's a delicious salad with nothing more added to it,' Becker says.

A smooth, filling vegetable soup Fill a saucepan with water, add a head of chopped cauliflower, a couple of chopped leeks and a clove of garlic. Cover the pan and boil the water until the cauliflower is tender. Cool slightly and transfer the soup to a blender. Add some salt, a touch of olive oil and a pinch of curry powder. Purée and serve.

A no-bread sandwich Sauté boneless chicken breast with ginger, garlic, chopped spring onions and soy sauce. Then wrap it in a large lettuce leaf. 'Sprinkle on some toasted cashews or peanuts, and it's even better,' Becker says.

them. As a side dish, serve tzatziki, made with 240g of strained Greek yoghurt, several cloves of diced garlic, half a peeled, shredded or diced cucumber, 1 tablespoon of olive oil, 2 teaspoons of lemon juice and chopped mint to taste. Put out warmed whole-grain flat bread or pitta bread and top it off with a glass of red wine or unsweetened iced tea. Eating Mediterranean-style is good for your heart and may improve insulin resistance.

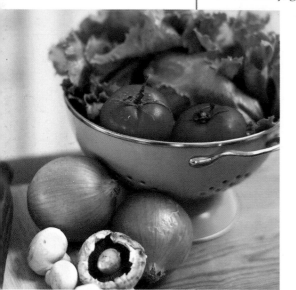

Make a big salad on Sunday. Lettuce and most crisp vegetables will remain fresh for several days in the refrigerator, so making a big salad on Sunday should last well into the week. Start with some diced carrots, celery, green beans, fresh broccoli and cauliflower florets. Add your favourite greens and store in an airtight container. Anything that contains moisture, such as tomatoes, cucumbers, olives, low-fat cheese, chicken, tuna or turkey, should be added just before serving.

Prepare for tomorrow the night before. Take 20 minutes from your evening TV viewing to do some preparation work that will make the next day go smoothly. Hard-boil eggs for breakfast and put them in the fridge, set the breakfast table, cut up fruit for your cereal or prepare a smoothie to chill in the refrigerator. Planning a berry crumble for dinner on Friday night? On Thursday make the crumble topping and seal it in a plastic bag or air-tight container. The next day you'll simply have to put it all together with the berries (or fruit) and bake.

Buy a whiteboard to track your portions of fibre-rich foods. Getting more fibre into your diet is one of the best ways to shrink your waistline and lower your blood glucose, but it's probably not on your mind when you're looking for something to eat. The answer? Every day, write down every fibre-rich food that passes your lips: your morning bowl of porridge (adding fruit or linseeds on top counts as one extra fibre food), your sandwich on two pieces of wholemeal bread (that counts as two) your afternoon apple, your side dishes of brown rice and steamed spinach at dinner. Aim for at least eight. The visual reminder will spur you on to eat more servings as the day progresses if you see you're falling short. Need one last serving after dinner? Snack on microwave popcorn in the evening.

Make breakfast count

Breakfast sounds like the easiest meal of the day, and in fact it is. It's also your best chance to increase the fibre in your diet, since the menu includes so many high-fibre choices like porridge and whole-grain cereal. And it's an excellent opportunity to get at least one serving of fruit (what's better on top of that porridge or cereal?) and one serving of dairy foods (what else would you pour onto your cereal but milk?). A bonus to eating breakfast is that it kick-starts your metabolism again after a night of fasting.

Eat breakfast at home. There's no reason to avoid restaurants altogether, but there is one meal you should always try to eat at home – and that's breakfast. Just consider some of the café alternatives: grilled sausage with bacon, scrambled egg, beans and toast can contain nearly 1,000kcal with 58g of fat and 51g of carbohydrate. A wholemeal bap with bacon may contain 571kcal, 23.7g of fat and 50g of carbohydrate, while a tempting large pecan Danish pastry has 428kcal, 26g fat and 51g carbohydrate. Compare those with a homemade bowl of porridge (40g) with 125ml skimmed milk, which contains just 12g of carbohydrates, 195kcal and 3g of fat.

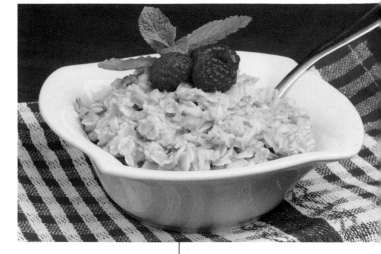

Always top your cereal with fruit. First, make sure that you're eating a cereal that contains at least 5g of fibre per serving. (Studies have found that people who regularly eat whole-grain cereal gain less weight than people who don't.) Make it even more diabetes-friendly by adding a handful of strawberries or blueberries.

Sprinkle 1 or 2 tablespoons of ground linseed on hot and cold cereal and yoghurt. Rich in protein and fibre, these tiny seeds are a godsend to your blood glucose as well as your heart. They also contain fatty acids that the body uses to make the same type of omega-3 fatty acids you get from fish. Like fish, the seeds lower cholesterol and help guard against inflammation. Plus their slightly nutty taste is delicious! Store whole seeds in the fridge and grind the amount you need with a spice or coffee grinder.

Have porridge several days a week, especially in winter. Porridge is one of the best breakfasts you can eat if you have diabetes. It contains 4g of fibre per serving, which will help to keep blood glucose levels steady. And studies have shown that eating a 50g serving of porridge five or six times a week can lower the risk of developing Type 2 diabetes by 39 per cent. Porridge may also

golden rule

Always eat breakfast

Even if your blood glucose is high in the morning, don't miss breakfast. Research shows that forgoing a morning meal increases the risk for obesity and insulin resistance. And studies confirm that breakfast eaters are better able to resist fatty and high-calorie foods later in the day. Aim to eat your breakfast at a similar time every morning, since keeping your blood glucose levels steady means eating consistently from day to day.

help you to eat less later in the day. One study found that people who ate porridge in the morning ate 30 per cent fewer calories at lunch compared with people who ate sugary, flaked cereal for breakfast.

Cook a large batch of coarse-cut oatmeal on Sunday mornings. Enjoy one serving and then refrigerate the rest. On weekday mornings, simply reheat in the microwave. Add raisins and cinnamon if you like. This saves time because fibre-rich coarse oatmeal can take up to 50 minutes to cook.

Make your own flavoured porridge. Instead of buying packets of flavoured porridge, which usually contain added sugar and salt and use more-processed oats, make your own porridge with a few flavour boosters – and diabetes busters! Start with old-fashioned or steel-cut oats and add chopped apples or peaches for sweetness (and fibre).

Go to work on an egg. When researchers studied 10,000 women, they found that the more calcium and vitamin D the women consumed, the less likely they were to have metabolic syndrome, a cluster of symptoms that increases the risk of diabetes and heart disease. Eggs are a good source of vitamin D (but, be sure to have them boiled or poached rather than fried), and include some dairy products, too, such as yoghurt and skimmed milk, as these are excellent sources of calcium. There is also some evidence to suggest that including low-fat dairy products can help people to lose weight.

Choose plain or diet yoghurts rather than low-fat or normal varieties. You can save 10–15g of carbohydrate this way.

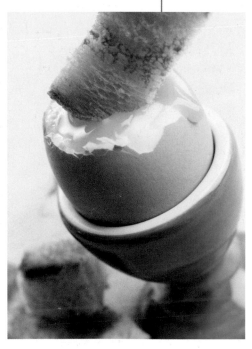

Low-fat yoghurt is not always best as manufacturers usually add extra sugar. You can save 50kcal by choosing a diet yoghurt instead of a low-fat variety.

Have an orange instead of orange juice. Juice is a source of concentrated carbohydrates and lacks the fibre of the whole fruit. The fruit will make you feel more satisfied and full.

When you drink juice, use a real juice glass. It's just 120ml. Fill it with orange juice, which contains 12g of carbohydrates, instead of grape juice, which contains 16g of carbs.

Doctor your tea or coffee with cinnamon. One way to get more blood-sugar-lowering cinnamon is to add a cinnamon stick to tea, or make a cinnamon tea by stirring a cinnamon stick in a cup of hot water. Or add half a teaspoon of powdered cinnamon to ground coffee before starting the pot.

Reinvent your lunch

You plan your dinners (hopefully), but lunch is all too often an afterthought. No problem. Like breakfast, lunch is a pretty simple meal to prepare. If you follow a sensible guidelines, it will take you a long way towards getting the foods that will help you to control your diabetes – and keep you full at least until it's time for a small, mid-afternoon snack. Your goal: include plenty of fibre (from salads, bean soups or wholemeal sandwich bread), vegetables and at least one source of lean protein (such as tuna or grilled chicken).

Swap the full-fat cheese slices in your sandwich for avocado slices. Yes, dairy foods are especially important if you have diabetes, but cheese has a shortcoming: it's full of saturated fat, which makes blood glucose control more difficult by making insulin sensitivity worse. Avocados, on the other hand, are high in mono-unsaturated fats, which help you to control your blood glucose and protect your heart. Their creamy richness mimics that of cheese. You don't need to eliminate cheese from your diet completely, just choose cheeses that taste good in lower-fat forms, such as low-fat mozzarella.

Fill up sandwiches with vegetables. There's nothing wrong with two slices of lean lunch meat such as roast turkey or ham in your sandwich, but most shop-bought sandwiches contain at least twice that much meat, not to mention all that mayonnaise and cheese. Make your sandwich at home (or go to a sandwich shop that will make it to your specifications), keep the meat lean (no salami or pepperoni) and modest, and pile on the vegetables. Don't stop at lettuce and tomato. Other great sandwich ingredients include sliced cucumber, onion, bean sprouts and roasted red or yellow peppers.

Add a smear of hummus. It's another fantastic sandwich filler and a great way to eat your pulses. Spread it onto a salad or chicken sandwich for extra protein and fibre. To make your own hummus, pour a can of chickpeas into your blender or food processor and add a tablespoon of olive oil and two cloves of chopped garlic. Add lemon juice to taste. Blend and enjoy. Traditionally, hummus is

make the change

The habit: Eating at least three daily servings of whole grains.

The results: Lower blood glucose levels and a lower risk of metabolic syndrome and heart disease.

The evidence: In one study of more than 750 men and women aged over 60, those who ate about three servings of whole grains a day were 54 per cent less likely to have metabolic syndrome, had lower fasting blood glucose levels and less body fat, and suffered 52 per cent fewer fatal heart attacks than people who ate less than one serving a day.

A serving of whole grains is one slice of wholemeal bread, 75g of whole-wheat pasta, or a 75g serving of brown rice, bulghur, barley or other whole grain.

made with tahini, a paste made from ground sesame seeds, but it's not necessary (and it adds a lot of fat). Keep your portion size to about 2 or 3 tablespoons of hummus.

Use oily fish on salads and in sandwiches. Herrings and sardines contain all-important healthy omega-3 fatty acids, which fight inflammation and help to prevent disease. But make sure you buy oily fish packed in brine, water or a tomato-based sauce, not oil. For example, 75g of herring fillets in tomato sauce contains 131kcal and 1.7g of saturated fat, whereas 75g of mackerel in an oil dressing contains 234kcal and 3.5g saturated fat.

Spread some mustard, not mayonnaise. Mustard has none of the fat contained in mayonnaise. A tablespoon of mustard has about 11kcal compared to 100kcal in the same amount of mayonnaise.

Add fruit to greens. Sneak in a serving of fruit with your salad. Toss slices of oranges, grapefruit, nectarines, apples, strawberries or blueberries to salads dressed with a vinaigrette and, for a protein boost, sprinkle with toasted almonds.

Fill up on lentils. Among legumes, lentils are some of the richest in protein. If you're not already eating them, open a can of lentil soup and enjoy a small bowl with your salad or sandwich. Or add a lentil salad to just about any lunch or dinner. Lentils cook quickly and you don't need to soak them first. Their soluble fibre content allows them to be digested slowly, so they have a blunting effect on your blood glucose.

Have a salad topped with rinsed canned beans. A large salad at lunch can knock off several vegetable servings in one go, but don't forget to add protein to keep you feeling full longer. Beans add the perfect bulk – both protein and fibre – to your lunch. Try kidney beans, chickpeas or black beans (especially good if you're adding avocado to your salad).

Buy a toasted sandwich maker or panini press. Sometimes a hot sandwich is more satisfying than a cold one, even if it contains the same number of calories. These grills toast sandwiches nicely and melt any cheese you've added. Try cooked chicken breast with tomato and spinach (add a little low-fat mozzarella if you like) or lean, reduced-salt ham and low-fat Brie. Buy a grill with removable nonstick grill plates to make cleaning easy.

Make dinner more diabetes friendly

If your diet is key to beating diabetes, your dinners are the cornerstone. Here's where most of us go overboard on calories, carbohydrates and fat. That doesn't mean you have to stick to rabbit food. Your dinners can be tasty and satisfying without wreaking havoc with your blood glucose. Here are some ways to do it.

Make a deal with your partner. The idea of preparing a meal, washing the dishes and cleaning the kitchen can quickly make you lose motivation when it comes to cooking a healthy meal. But before you give up on your eating plan and decide to have frozen pizza, tell your partner that you'll cook if he or she will do the cleaning. You'll both benefit from the home-cooked meal, and you'll be able to put your feet up afterwards.

Cook once, eat twice. Make double the amount and you'll have dinner for tomorrow. Or pack it up and freeze it for a day when you don't have time to cook.

Make a pot of tea before you start cooking. Cooks nibble. It's unconscious and it's incessant. You can consume several hundred calories in no time tasting the soup, sampling the roast, stealing a little cheese, nibbling while you wait for the water to boil. Controlling this is critical for people who cook regularly – and that should include you. One way to curtail this bad habit is to brew a pot of tea before you even begin cooking so you can turn to your mug instead of your food while you cook.

Start with a simple salad. You'll eat less of the main meal and take in more vegetables to boot. Dress it with a splash of vinegar or lemon juice or an olive oil vinaigrette – not a creamy dressing.

whip it together!

Garlicky green beans

With this master recipe, you can take all kinds of vegetables and infuse them with the heady aroma of garlic and onions. For instance, try broccoli, cauliflower, sliced asparagus or sliced red peppers in place of the green beans.

Steam 450g trimmed **green beans** for 5 minutes over boiling water. Remove from the heat and put the green beans into a bowl of **iced water** to refresh. Drain again and set aside. In a medium pan, heat 2 teaspoons **olive oil**. Add 1 small diced **onion** and 3 finely chopped **garlic cloves** and sauté for 3 minutes. Add 1 tin (400g) chopped **tomatoe**s and the steamed green beans. Cook for 2 minutes.

Use your vegetable of the week. In the supermarket chapter we suggested you designate a vegetable of the week. Don't let it rot in your fridge. If it's bok choy, add a handful to soup (homemade or from a tin) on Monday; sauté it with garlic and 1 teaspoon olive oil on Tuesday; chop it small and add to spaghetti sauce on Wednesday; mix it into a stir-fry on Thursday; and try it on pizza (with a whole-wheat crust) on Friday. If you juice, add both the stalk and the leaves to your juicer and drink for its vitamin C and fibre content.

Go vegetarian at least once a week. You'll get much more fibre and far less saturated fat. Instead of meat lasagna, have vegetable lasagna using aubergine or a mix of vegetables such as broccoli, carrots, peppers, mushrooms and courgettes. Likewise, vegetable chilli is a perfectly tasty alternative to meat chilli.

Replace a liquid with a spray. Take any food that's typically fried in butter or oil and brown it in a nonstick frying pan with a little cooking spray instead. Cooking spray can be substituted for oil whenever you fry. It takes a little getting used to – you will need to watch the pan closely – but you will save yourself lots of calories and fat without losing flavour.

Savour the crunch of oven-baked chicken and chips. Put fried chicken and chips back on the menu without overloading on saturated fat. Dip strips of boneless, skinless chicken into a little flour, coat in beaten egg, yoghurt or skimmed milk, and cover with plain breadcrumbs mixed with herbs. Then bake in the oven at 180°C for 20 to 30 minutes. The chicken will have a crispy coating that satisfies your taste for fried chicken. For the chips, cut white or sweet potatoes into strips, soak in water for 20 minutes and spread on a baking sheet. Drizzle with olive oil, sprinkle with salt and pepper, and bake for 40 minutes at 180°C, turning halfway through.

When beef is on the menu, choose lean cuts. These include filet mignon, sirloin and fillet steak. Always trim off any visible fat. A serving of meat is no more than 75g cooked, 100g raw.

Put your meals on a bed of greens. Chefs everywhere are serving this or that dish on a bed of greens. You can do the same thing: simply steam some spinach, kale or

golden rule

Fill half your plate with vegetables

If you want to see a nice full plate in front of you, fill half of it with non-starchy vegetables (that means no potatoes or sweetcorn). Split the other half between a protein, such as roasted chicken, and a starch, such as 75g of brown rice. That gives you two servings of vegetables and ensures that you don't overdo it on starchy carbohydrates. Add a side salad and now you have three vegetable servings in your meal.

Swiss chard, then put it on your plate and lay your fish or chicken on top. When you grow tired of dark leafy greens, get creative and make your 'bed' out of steamed mangetout, sugarsnap peas, and sprouts such as alfalfa or or mung bean.

Top fish or chicken with fruit salsa. Using salsa is an exciting way to sneak in a serving of fruit and give simple dishes flavour without fat. Make a fruity salsa by combining chunks of pineapple, mango or papaya with chopped onions, ginger, garlic, mint, coriander and hot chilli flakes. Let it sit for 30 minutes at room temperature or up to 4 hours in the fridge.

Make a fruit glaze to drizzle over fish. Try this simple American recipe from Deborah Carabet, chef and nutritionist in Los Angeles, California: to a saucepan add 60ml of orange juice or water, puréed mango (canned) and a handful of frozen or fresh mango chunks. Heat over medium heat until it forms a sweet glaze. Drizzle over grilled salmon or other fish.

Lay thick slices of pineapple or peach on the grill. Brush them first with a little olive oil so they don't stick. Fruit has never tasted so good. You can even serve these for dessert.

Have a main dish salad once a week and ring the changes. If you put the same old vegetables in your salad every week, sooner or later you may be more inclined to toss it into the bin than savour every bite. Get out of the rut by trying new ingredients, such as sweetfire mini beetroot or artichoke hearts from a can, sweet piquant peppers (from a jar), chicory leaves, beansprouts or sautéed varieties of exotic mushrooms. Include a protein food such as beans or grilled chicken breast.

whip it together!

Tropical fruit salsa

This hot and sweet salsa, loaded with vitamin C, adds an extra-special finish to grilled chicken or fish.

150g fresh chopped **pineapple** or **mango**

1 **kiwi**, peeled and diced

1 small **orange**, peeled and diced

1 teaspoon deseeded and finely chopped **red chilli**

1 tablespoon finely chopped **red onion**

1 tablespoon finely chopped **red pepper**

1 tablespoon fresh **lime juice**

1 teaspoon **sugar** or **sugar substitute**

Combine all the ingredients in a bowl. Cover and refrigerate 1 hour. Serve with grilled chicken or fish. For extra flavour, sprinkle on 1 tablespoon of chopped fresh coriander, mint or parsley.

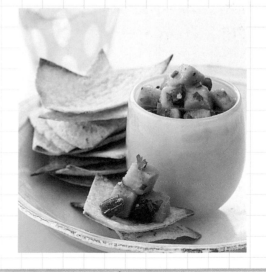

Carbohydrate counting

Because carbohydrates (carbs) raise blood glucose, managing them successfully is key to managing your diabetes. One way to do it is through carbohydrate counting. Knowing how many carbs you can have throughout the day – and following those guidelines consistently every day – will set your blood glucose levels on an even keel, make you feel more energised, and help you to avoid the complications of diabetes.

Most of the foods you eat – from milk and fruit to breads and cereal – contain carbohydrates. You can't avoid them, and you wouldn't want to. Carbohydrates are your main fuel source.. The trick is to avoid eating too many in one day or at one sitting. When you eat carbohydrates, your body breaks the food down into glucose, which enters the bloodstream. That triggers your pancreas to release the hormone insulin, which helps to move the glucose into your cells where it can be used as energy. The more carbohydrates you eat, the more insulin your body needs to help convert the food to energy.

When you have diabetes, your pancreas doesn't produce enough insulin or your body can't use the insulin to move the glucose into the cells. Starved cells make you feel tired and sluggish. Chronically high blood glucose levels boost the production of free radicals and lower your immunity, on top of other negative effects. The key is to gain better control over your blood glucose levels by learning just how many carbohydrates you should eat throughout the day. Here's what to do.

1 Calculate your energy needs

The amount of calories we need to stay healthy varies with age and how heavy we are. Using the table (above, right), insert your weight in kilograms to determine the number of calories you need each day to maintain your weight.

Age (years)	Female
18–29	14.8 x weight (kg) + 487
30–59	8.3 x weight (kg) + 846
60+	9.1 x weight (kg) + 658

Age (years)	Male
18–29	15.1 x weight (kg) + 692
30–59	11.5 x weight (kg) + 873
60+	11.7 x weight (kg) + 587

2 Determine your activity level factor

Now you need to take into account how active you are. This is based on your gender and your level of physical activity. The more active you are, the more calories – and carbohydrates – you can eat. If you're a couch potato, rate yourself 'sedentary'. If you exercise occasionally, rate yourself 'lightly active'. If you exercise regularly, you're 'active'. If you exercise strenuously almost every day, you're 'very active'.

Activity Level	Female	Male
sedentary	1.4	1.4
lightly active	1.5	1.5
active	1.6	1.7
very active	2.1	1.8

Multiply your answer from section 1 with the activity factor from section 2 to find your daily energy needs.

Number of calories x activity level = daily calorie needs

To lose 0.5kg a week, you'll need a calorie reduction of around 600kcal per day from your estimated calorie needs. But women shouldn't eat fewer than 1,200kcal a day and men fewer than 1,500kcal a day unless under supervision of a registered dietitian.

3 Determine how many carbohydrates you need

The chart below assumes that you need 50 per cent of your calories from carbohydrates. (Work with a registered dietitian to determine the best carbohydrate targets for you. Diabetes UK and the British Dietetic Association recommend that 40–60 per cent of your total calories should come from carbohydrates.)

Carb portions are foods with about 10g of carbohydrates per serving. For example, 200ml milk has 10g of carbohydrates and would count as one carb portion. Carbohydrate content is usually listed on a food's nutrition label.

Calories	Carbs	Carb portions
1,200	150	15
1,500	190	19
1,800	220	22
2,000	250	25
2,200	275	27
2,400	300	30
2,800	350	35
3,000	375	37
3,200	400	40
3,400	425	42

4 Spread your carb portions throughout your meals

If you want to eat 5 carb portions for breakfast, you could have 100ml of orange juice (1 carb portion), 2 slices of granary toast (3 carb portions), 2 teaspoons of marmalade (1 carb portion) and a cup of fruit tea (no portions).

5 Check your blood glucose

Check your blood glucose before a meal and 2 hours after it, noting the results and what you ate. This will help you to find out what works best for you throughout the day, as we all respond differently to the amount of carbohydrate eaten. You won't have to check your blood glucose every day for ever, but do it for several days to get a feel for how your body responds to your meals. Diabetes UK recommends that blood glucose levels should fall within these ranges:

Fasting or before your meal:
4.0–6.0 mmol/l

Two hours after the start of your meal:
less than 10mmol/l

6 Make adjustments

If your blood glucose levels are too high 2 hours after a meal, try getting some exercise or adjusting what you eat. Take a walk after eating to see if the levels go down, or trying taking out a carb portion. If that doesn't work, consult your health-care professional. Perhaps a medication adjustment will help.

7 Stay consistent

Eat your meals at around the same time every day. Skipping meals or varying the amount of carbohydrates you eat at different meals from day to day will make it harder for you to control your blood glucose levels.

Try a new shape. Buy pre-cut vegetables or cut them yourself into new shapes and you may find that you want to eat more of them. Carrot sticks have a crunch that makes you feel a little like you're eating potato crisps. Cut courgettes, green or yellow, into long strips and grill. Imagine they're chips.

Use quinoa instead of white rice. Quinoa raises blood glucose less than rice does (assuming you eat the amount of barley that you'd eat of rice), so consider it your new rice. Serve it with stir-fried vegetables, add it to soups and stews, toss it into your bean salad, or make it as a side dish. High in soluble fibre, it's a lot like porridge in the way it reduces cholesterol levels and the risk of heart disease.

Savour the sweetness of roasted vegetables. Bring out the sweetness of veggies such as aubergine, onions, peppers, courgettes and squash by brushing them with olive oil, sprinkling with salt and pepper, and roasting in a 200°C oven until soft. Add firm vegetables such as aubergine, onions and peppers to the grill for 10 to 15 minutes. For softer or smaller vegetables like sliced courgettes, tomatoes and carrots, use a grilling basket or foil parcel and cook for 6 to 8 minutes.

Use vegetables as fillers. Don't confine vegetables just to the side of your plate. Throw in a couple of handfuls of frozen peas and carrots to your rice or couscous during the last five minutes of cooking. Add chopped onions and spinach to meat loaf or hamburgers made with lean beef. Stir chopped peppers and mushrooms into canned or bottled spaghetti sauce. Add cooked kale, mushrooms and onions to stuffing. Rub the fuzziness off the stalks of okra, slice and add to soups, stews and casseroles.

For extra flavour, steam vegetables in chicken stock. Instead of adding water to your steamer or saucepan, add chicken or vegetable stock. You'll add flavour without fat to carrots, courgettes, cauliflower, sugarsnap peas and other vegetables.

Save the water from steaming. After steaming your vegetables, pour the water into a covered jar and keep it in the fridge to use for stock the next time you make soup. The antioxidants from vegetables help stave off complications from diabetes, including problems with kidneys and eyes, and they may even help prevent the disease in the first place. Throw away if you have not used it after a couple of days.

Think bean filling for your Mexican enchiladas. The next time you have a Mexican meal, skip the beef or chicken and fill your enchiladas and tacos with beans (not refried). For an easy meal of enchiladas, drain and rinse tinned cannellini beans and add them to a pan with onions, mushrooms and other vegetables. Add some enchilada sauce and serve in whole-wheat tortillas with low-fat cheese.

Toss a 5 minute bean salad. Choose three or four kinds of tinned beans – such as black, kidney, butter, black-eyed or borlotti – and drain and rinse well to get rid of some of the salt. Then toss with chopped red onion, red pepper and some vinaigrette-style salad dressing. Use a tablespoon of dressing per 100g bean salad.

Replace white potatoes with sweet potatoes. Sweet potatoes raise blood glucose less than white potatoes do. If the sweet potato is large, cut in half and share one potato between two people. Be sure to eat the skin for its fibre.

Add wine or vinegar to strawberries. Take 100g of hulled strawberries and drizzle with balsamic vinegar or soak in white wine for a sweet, indulgent-tasting dessert that satisfies about 75 per cent of your daily vitamin C requirement. And like other berries, strawberries contain powerful antioxidants that help to protect your body from the ravages of high blood glucose.

Have fruit for dessert. Fruit is, after all, nature's sweetmeat. So on those nights when you eat dessert (we suggest once or twice a week), try a roasted plum, 75g of berries with yoghurt on top, or fruit crumble (go heavy on the fruit, oats and cinnamon and very light on the sugar and butter).

'Bake' an apple in your microwave. Just core an apple, sprinkle the inside with cinnamon and a touch of sugar, and microwave for 3 minutes or until soft.

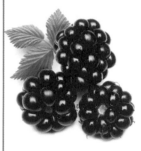

PLUS POINT
Berries contain powerful antioxidants that help to protect your body from the ravages of high blood glucose.

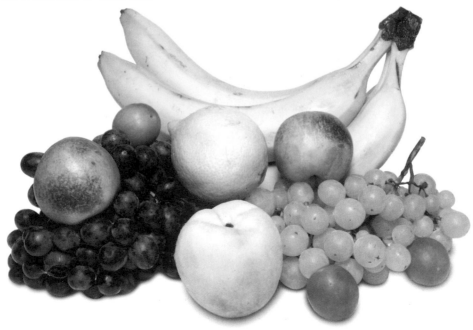

Diabetes-friendly snacks

There's some traditional dietary advice, such as 'Don't eat between meals', that you might want to take with a pinch of salt. If you go more than 4 or 5 hours between meals, a mid-afternoon snack might be just what the doctor ordered to help you to keep your blood glucose steady. Snacking is also important if you're taking medication that could cause a blood-sugar low between meals. Discuss with a health professional which snacking approach is right for you.

Keep your snacks to 150kcal or less. The danger of snacks is that they can become more like extra meals if you go overboard. First, make sure you're truly hungry – and not just bored or stressed or craving chocolate – before reaching for a snack. Then limit yourself to 150kcal per snack. This will help to keep your snacking 'honest'. After all, it's hard to find a chocolate bar with only 150kcal. And if you're hankering after chocolate, and a healthier snack doesn't appeal, you're probably not truly hungry.

Beware of low-fat snacks. Studies show that people tend to eat about 28 per cent more of a snack if they think it's low-fat. But low-fat snacks are not necessarily low in sugar, and tend to have only 11 per cent fewer calories than their full-fat counterparts. Stick to the same amount you'd eat if you thought the snack was full-fat.

Put your snacks on a plate. Eat straight out of the bag and you're guaranteed to eat more, whether it's crisps, sweets or biscuits. Instead, put a small portion on a plate, seal up the bag and put it away. Then sit down and enjoy your snack.

Have a bag full. A single serving bag, that is. You're much more likely to stop after one serving if you don't have to measure it out yourself. If paying more for extra packaging that will eventually clog landfills bothers you, separate your snacks yourself into reusable single-serving containers when you get home from the supermarket. They'll be ready to grab when you're ready to eat them.

Eat a handful of nuts. Almonds, walnuts, pecans, peanuts and cashews contain the healthy monounsaturated fats that lower cholesterol and reduce the risk of heart disease. And because they're packed with protein and 'good' fat, they won't raise blood glucose as much as savoury crackers or pretzels do. Because many nuts are high in calories (almonds are the lowest), stick to 25g, or about the amount that will fit in the palm of your hand.

Try a few whole-grain crackers with peanut butter. They contain more protein and fewer carbohydrates than a bigger pile of crackers on their own, and your blood glucose won't rise as much.

PLUS POINT
Nuts are packed with protein and 'good' fat so they don't raise blood glucose nearly as much as savoury crackers.

Snack on raw vegetables. Get in an extra serving of vegetables by nibbling on cherry tomatoes, carrots, red and green peppers, cucumbers, broccoli and cauliflower. Eat them plain or dip them in low-fat yoghurt, a light salad dressing or hummus (stick with 1 to 2 tablespoons' worth).

Spread some tomato salsa over aubergine slices. The salsa has only about 15g of carbohydrates, 80kcal and 1g of fat.

Sip a small cup of vegetable soup. Cook nonstarchy vegetables such as spinach, onion, celery, green beans and squash in some vegetable or chicken stock. It's filling, full of nutrients and low in carbohydrates.

Indulge in a few decadent bites. Have a snack of three dried apricots, a small piece – one or two squares – of dark chocolate and three walnuts or almonds, suggests Vicki Saunders, RD, who teaches nutrition education programmes at St Helena Hospital in Napa Valley, California. Savour every nibble.

Blend a fruit smoothie. Combine half a chopped banana, 170ml low-fat plain yoghurt and a sweetener. Blend until smooth.

Freeze grapes and peeled bananas. Seal them in a sandwich bag and throw it into the freezer. Once frozen, they're a refreshing and healthy treat. You can eat 20 red seedless grapes and still consume only 100kcal.

Eat an apple – and the skin. An apple with the skin contains about 3g of fibre. The skin packs a double benefit, carrying healthy soluble fibre that helps to lower cholesterol and prevent heart disease as well as antioxidants that fight free radicals and lower the risk of diabetes complications.

Try low-fat mini cheeses. Each one contains only 50kcal. These are one of the few portable goodies rich in sugar-steadying protein.

Have your chocolate 'bar' frozen. By that we mean enjoy a frozen chocolate milk stick. They taste delightfully chocolatey but contain only about 80kcal.

Freeze berries and fruit for use in smoothies. Make up single portion mixed bags of chopped banana, apple and berries that you can keep in the freezer. Take one out, allow to thaw a little, then blend with 200ml soya milk for a cool smoothie.

whip it together!

Cheesy courgette bites

When you're hankering for a tasty, cheesy snack, pop these in the oven and enjoy a low-carbohydrate, healthy treat.

Cut a **courgette** into 2cm thick slices and scoop out some of the inside flesh. Add ½ teaspoon crumbled **blue cheese**, top with a **tomato** slice, a sprinkle of **Parmesan cheese**, **basil** and **pepper**. Bake at 200°C for 5–7 minutes, or until the cheese is melted. One courgette bite has only 1g of carbohydrate, 19kcal and 1g of fat.

>> continued on page 61

Kitchen workout

Have you ever thought of taking a spot of exercise while you wait for water to boil or the roast to come out of the oven? With the help of a straight-backed kitchen chair, you can become more flexible, with a greater range of motion in no time flat. You may even feel calmer and more relaxed afterwards – and be less likely to overeat at dinner.

1 Arm lift

Sit in the chair and extend your arms to either side at shoulder height, palms facing forward. Slowly, over the space of 5 seconds, raise your arms until your hands meet over your head.

   Hold this position for 5 seconds, and then spend 5 more seconds returning your arms to the original position. Repeat five more times.

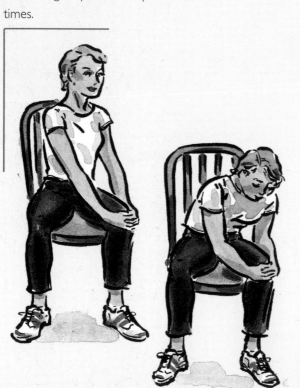

2 Back stretch

Sit in a chair, with your feet flat on the floor. Lace the fingers of your hands together and place them across the front of your right knee.

   Lean as far towards your left knee as you can, breathing out as you do, and then return to an upright position. Spend 3 seconds leaning forward and 3 seconds returning. Repeat four times, then switch sides.

3 Leg lift

Sit with your feet flat on the floor. Slowly, over the space of 5 seconds, lift your left leg until it extends straight forward. Hold for 5 seconds, then slowly lower it back down. Repeat nine more times, then change legs.

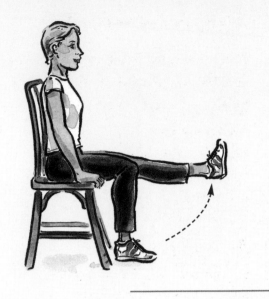

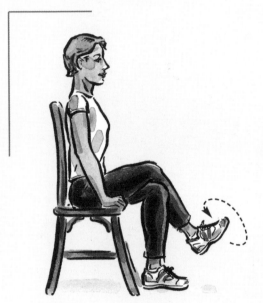

4 Foot circles

While sitting, cross your right leg over your left knee. Over a period of 4 seconds, move your right foot to the right and draw a large circle. Repeat nine times, then switch feet.

5 Quarter squat

Stand behind the chair and place your hands on the top of the chair back. Squat slightly, lowering your hips about 10cm, making sure your knees don't extend beyond your toes. Spend 2 seconds lowering your body and 2 seconds standing erect again. Repeat seven more times.

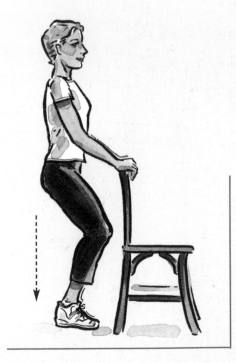

>> continued on page 60

6 Knee lift

Turn sideways to the chair back and place your left hand on the chair back.

Keeping your back straight, slowly raise your right knee as high as it will go, then slowly lower it again. Still holding the chair back with your left hand, perform the exercise with your left leg. Do the exercise five times with each leg.

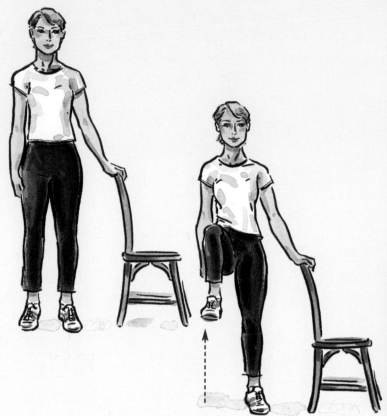

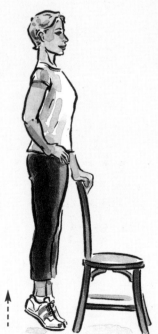

7 Heel raise

Stand behind the chair with your feet 10cm apart, your left hand on the chair back and your right hand on your hip. Raise onto your toes over 2 seconds, and then lower back down over 2 seconds. Repeat nine more times.

Special mission: curb your carbohydrates

Too many of the carbohydrates we eat today are the kind that raise blood glucose too high and too fast. They include rolls, biscuits, white bread and other baked goods made with white flour, easily digested starches such as potatoes and refined grains such as white rice. Eating too many of these foods increases insulin resistance and makes it harder to control your blood glucose. So here are some ideas to help you to cut down.

Avoid rolls at dinner time. Bread isn't bad for you, especially if it's wholemeal. But if you had a sandwich at lunch or toast with your eggs at breakfast, that's probably all the bread you need for the day.

Swap the tortilla for a lettuce-leaf wrap. Wrap the lettuce around canned tuna or salmon, shredded carrots, diced celery and pepper slices for a delicious and healthy snack.

Hold your sandwich together with aubergine slices instead of bread. Grill the aubergine until brown, then add slices of low-fat mozzarella and tomato.

Mash cauliflower instead of potatoes. Add some steamed cauliflower to your blender and purée with enough skimmed milk to make it velvety. Drizzle with olive oil and season with salt and pepper.

Make cauliflower 'rice'. Using a food processor, shred your cauliflower until its texture resembles rice, then lightly steam. Add the cauliflower 'rice' to recipes that call for cooked rice.

Indulge in parsnip and carrot 'chips'. Cut down the length of parsnips and carrots to make long, thin strips of the vegetables. Place on a baking sheet, drizzle with olive oil, sprinkle with salt and pepper, and roast in a 200°C oven for about 40 minutes.

Replace potato salad with coleslaw. Coleslaw makes a great side dish – cabbage is low in calories and high in fibre. For the dressing, whisk together 160ml fat-free sour cream, 160ml plain low-fat yoghurt, 60ml cider vinegar, 1 tablespoon of low-fat mayonnaise and 4 teaspoons sugar. Toss with a red and a green shredded cabbage, 50g blue cheese, 4 Granny Smith apples cut into wedges and 2 finely sliced red peppers.

Cut your pasta in half. Serve yourself 50g of pasta instead of 100g and bulk it up with sautéed peppers, mushrooms or other vegetables.

Feel a carbohydrate craving coming on? Drink a glass of water and wait 15 minutes. If you're still craving a particular food, put one serving on a plate and sit down at a table to eat it. When you've finished, get out of the kitchen. This habit will keep you from overeating without feeling deprived.

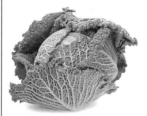

PLUS POINT
Cabbage is incredibly low in calories and high in fibre.

At the table

In general, people are on better eating behaviour when they're in public or with a group of friends or business associates. For example, you're less likely to finish off your meal in record time. When you're at home, practise these tips at the table to help yourself slow down, eat more moderate portions and even sneak in some extra vegetables.

Get out your best china. Smaller plates mean you'll naturally eat smaller meals and plates from the 1930s and 1940s were as small as 13–15cm in diameter. A typical plate today is 25–30cm across. If you'd rather save the china for special occasions, use side plates instead and save the dinner plates for company.

Banish the television from the kitchen and dining room. It's too easy to fall into mindless eating when you're in front of the TV. Another good reason not to watch: studies show that the more time people spend in front of the television, the more likely they are to be obese.

Hang a mirror beside your dining table. If you have to face yourself while you're eating, you'll find it harder to gorge on food or eat too fast. Also, dieters say that looking themselves in the eye reminds them of their goals.

Set a 30 minute timer as you take your first bite. Then don't take your last bite until it goes off. It takes about 20 minutes to feel full after eating, so taking it slowly will allow your brain to catch up with your stomach and turn off the urge to keep eating.

Limit 'help yourself' meals. Setting out a heaped plate of spaghetti and meatballs will only tempt you to overindulge, so serve it on individual plates and in moderate portions.

Encourage extra helpings of vegetables by serving them in a big bowl or platter. Vegetables are the exception to the rule above. No matter what vegetable you're serving for dinner, put out a lot and let people help themselves – and go back for seconds.

Put out a plate of raw vegetables. If your family tends to mill around the table just before dinner is served – or if you feel the need to nibble before the food hits the plates – have carrot sticks, cucumber slices, string beans, cherry tomatoes or any other types of raw vegetable out where everyone can easily reach them. Picking at them can substantially lower your consumption of the more calorie-dense main course.

Leave two bites on your plate. Follow this simple trick at lunch and dinner and you can save more than 100kcal a day.

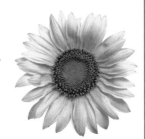

PLUS POINT
Dieters say that looking themselves in the eye reminds them of their goals.

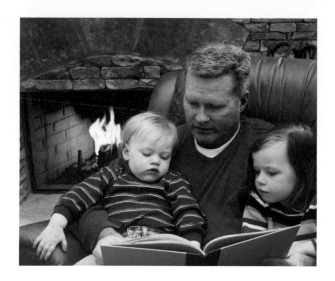

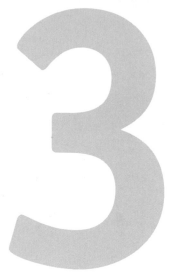

In your living room

As its name suggests, this is the room

where we spend most of our time –

the centre of our living space. Change

a habit here and there and maximise

your fun and your health.

Better TV: 'watching' your waistline

Few modern conveniences have done more to damage the health of humankind than the television. We barely move a muscle while we're glued to the screen, and images of fatty and sugary foods tempt us at every advert break. The next time you sit in front of the TV, keep these tips in mind.

Make a to-do list for commercial breaks. Ten minutes before the start of your favourite programme, make a list of five 2 minute jobs you can do during the adverts. Your list may include things like dusting the living-room blinds, sorting through the magazine rack or watering plants. Gather all of the materials you need for these projects and keep them at the ready. Accomplishing these little tasks will keep you moving around the house – and the distraction will keep you away from thoughts of food.

Hide your TV's remote control. Take a trip down memory lane, back to a time when televisions didn't have remote controls. Changing the channel and adjusting the volume used to get us all up and about, didn't it? So try taking the batteries out of your television's remote control and hiding it in a drawer or cupboard; that will get you off the sofa and on your feet. And while you're up and about, you may remember to do something else that will keep you active.

Pull the plug on 'TV dinners'. If you love having your dinner in the living room in front of the television news or a game show, break the habit. Studies suggest that the more TV people watch while eating, the fewer fruit and vegetables they consume. Researchers believe that this may happen because TV

golden rule

Do some exercise while watching TV

Use the time in front of the telly to get some exercise, even if it's mild exercise. Break out your elastic exercise bands (see page 214) to do some simple strength training, or – if you're sure you'll use it – buy an exercise bike and pedal away while you enjoy your programmes.
Or fold laundry – it's much better for your body (and your household) than being a couch potato.

programmes often feature unhealthy snacks or fattening food, which influences what the viewer then chooses to eat.

Keep your snack foods as far as possible from your sofa. Storing crisps, biscuits or other snacks anywhere near the television makes it far too easy to eat junk food without even thinking. If you store them at the back of the larder you'll at least have to climb up to get them – and passing the fruit bowl on the kitchen worktop may remind you that an apple would be a better snack.

Nibble on baked, not fried, crisps. If you are going to have crisps in the house – and occasionally nibble them in the evening – avoid regular salty potato crisps and switch to the baked variety. Whereas one serving of regular potato crisps contains 150kcal and 10g of fat, the same serving of the baked variety contains 110kcal and 1.5g of fat. It's not just crisps that are available baked – it's easy to find baked tortilla chips and other snacks, too. Just remember to eat no more than you would if the snacks were fried.

Brush your teeth after dinner. Some successful dieters say that tooth-brushing is their secret weapon to weight loss. Once you've eaten your evening meal, brush your teeth and enjoy the sensation of the fresh minty taste. You'll be less likely to mindlessly dig into a tub of ice cream or reach for a packet of biscuits while you're watching TV.

Keep your hands busy. Sometimes smoking or nibbling on fattening snacks becomes a habit because it keeps our hands busy. Put those idle hands to work by sorting out paperwork, model-making, needlework or knitting while you're on the sofa. The more engrossed you become in your pastime, the less likely you are to reach for a snack – and you won't want to scatter crumbs.

Delay your viewing hours. Scientists say that the more people watch TV, the more they eat. If you'd like to minimise the time you sit down viewing, here's a simple way to do it: study each night's TV

make the change

The habit: Watching less television.

The result: Lower body weight.

The evidence: Researchers from the United States Department of Agriculture surveyed more than 9,000 adults about their eating and television viewing habits. Adults who watched less than 1 hour of TV daily (only 15 per cent of those surveyed) consumed on average 1,896kcal per day, compared to 2,033kcal among those who watched more than 2 hours a day (nearly 60 per cent of those surveyed). What's more, the men in the second group were 22 per cent more likely to be overweight or obese than those in the first; the women in the second group were 36 per cent more likely to weigh too much. The study concluded that watching a lot of television or videos intrudes on time you might otherwise spend on physical activities. Also, people tend to consume more high-calorie snack foods while they're watching the TV.

whip it together!

Crispy cheese crisps

If you must have a snack in front of the TV, make it a healthy one. These treats have all the crunch that comes with crisps and biscuits – minus the guilt.

Cut two 20cm **whole-wheat tortillas** into 8 triangles. Coat a baking sheet with low-fat cooking spray. In a small bowl, combine 2 tablespoons **olive oil**, 1 finely chopped **garlic** clove and ½ teaspoon of dried **basil**. Brush this mixture over each of the wedges. Sprinkle a little grated **Parmesan cheese** over all wedges. Bake at 180°C for 8 to 9 minutes until toasted.

listings, identify one programme you would have watched, and record it for another day. Instead, go for a walk or cycle ride, or get your address book out and call a friend you haven't heard from in months. Exercise and social connection will do your body and soul much more good than a TV crime drama and the snacking that often goes with it.

Relax and laugh. If you're going to watch television after dinner, try to make it a comedy rather than a drama. Scientists in Japan made an interesting discovery: people with diabetes who laughed their way through a television comedy straight after a meal had lower blood glucose than people who watched a humdrum lecture.

Practise a new skill – juggling! This is mad enough to be fun. Stash three juggling balls or bags in a living-room cupboard. When you're watching a programme that doesn't require much concentration, pick up your juggling equipment and practise your toss-and-catch. Not only will you impress friends with your skilful party piece, but your clowning around will burn more than 270kcal per hour.

Keep resistance bands under the sofa. These stretchy latex bands, sold in sports shops and department stores, can give just about any part of your body a great workout even while you're watching TV. For a leg workout, tie one end to the sofa leg and the other to your ankle, then try to straighten your leg. Repeat 8 to 12 times, then switch legs. For more resistance band exercises, see page 214.

Watch a fitness show. If you like to watch TV, perhaps a 'reality' show where people are challenged to get fit or lose weight will inspire you? Better still, rent or buy an exercise video or DVD and pop it in. There are many choices of exercise (aerobics, Pilates, yoga, tai chi, belly dancing) for just about every fitness level – even seated workouts for those with mobility problems.

Get active in front of the screen. Delight your grandchildren and friends of any age by investing in a Nintendo Wii gaming console and accessories. You plug the console into your TV and mains, just like a DVD player, set up its sensor, put some batteries into the special Wii-mote (remote), and you're ready to play. The basic Wii package comes with a game disk called Wii Sports, which enables you to play tennis, baseball, bowling, golf and boxing interactively. What makes these games especially fun and different is that you actively 'play' the sports with the remote (the sensor bar inteprets your action on the screen), taking – according to the game – a golf swing, a tennis forehand or a throw of the bowling ball. Participants play with such energy that the manufacturers quickly fitted straps to the Wii-mote, to prevent it being accidentally thrown at the screen.

Hit the 'off' switch

Even better than being active while watching TV is turning it off altogether. There are plenty of other things you can do in your living room. Activities that allow you to interact with friends and family members – such as a lively game of cards – are easy ways to relax while keeping your mind working. And if you just can't be compelled to get off the sofa, why not at least invite your partner to join you? If your intimacy leads you to the bedroom, all the better: sex is a renowned stress reliever. One scientific study demonstrated that when couples have sex, their blood pressure returns to normal more quickly the next time they encounter a stressful situation – and the effect lasts for as much as a week.

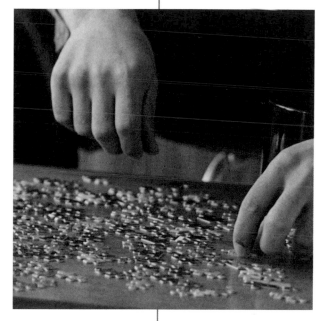

Create a games cabinet. Appoint yourself 'game master' and stock a shelf or cabinet with board games and other amusements. Set aside a night every week when you turn off the television, invite some friends round and play dominoes, Monopoly, Scrabble, poker or some other absorbing game. You'll get a mental workout, engage in some friendly competition and have some blood glucose-lowering laughs.

Put together an enormous jigsaw puzzle. There's something Zen-like in the quiet, contemplative process of slowly building a jigsaw puzzle. You turn your attention for hours to the minute detail

>> continued on page 70

Have a ball while exercising

They may look like giant toys, but stability balls, sold in most sports shops, provide a fun way to exercise indoors. The inflatable balls are used primarily to strengthen back and abdominal muscles, though they can also improve balance and flexibility. They're lightweight enough to stow away in a cupboard, but some people like the balls so much that they make them fixtures in the living room. Here are a few exercises to get you started.

1 Hip lift

Lie on your back on the floor, with your hands palms-down at your sides and your heels placed on the stability ball. Tighten your abdominal and buttock muscles as you slowly lift your hips into the air until your body makes a straight line. Hold for 3 seconds and slowly return to the starting position. Repeat a total of ten times.

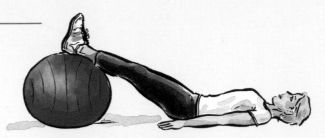

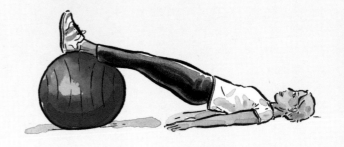

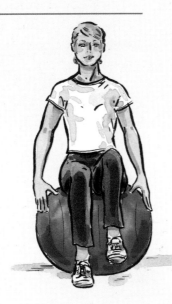

2 Balance challenge

Sit on top of the ball with your feet flat on the floor, hip-width apart. Place your hands on the ball at your sides. Hold your back straight and pull your abdominal muscles in. Now lift your left foot 15cm off the ground, hold it there for 5 seconds, and return to the starting position. Repeat with the right foot. Do the whole sequence five times.

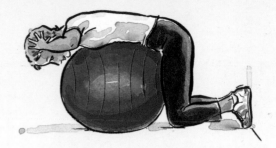

3 Back extension

Start on your knees, with your feet against a wall and the ball on the floor against the front of your legs. Lean forward onto the ball, raising your knees 10cm off the floor. Place your hands on either side of your head to the side of your head, fingertips near the temples and elbows straight out to the side.

Raise your upper body until your back is straight, pause, then lower your body again until your chest rests against the ball. Repeat a total of five times.

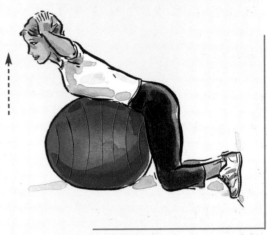

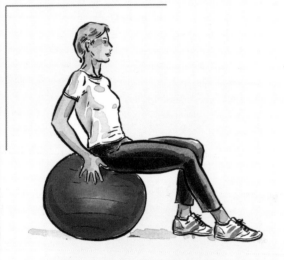

4 Forward walk

Sit on top of the ball with your feet flat on the floor. Place your hands on the ball for balance, or place one hand against a wall if you need the support.

Slowly step forward, letting the ball roll up your back until your shoulder blades are on top of the ball and your legs are bent at right angles. Slowly step back to the starting position. Repeat a total of three times.

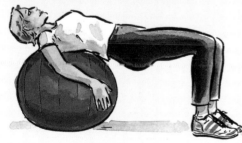

TRAINING TIP Choose the right ball for your height

If you're 1.5m (4ft 11in) to 1.6m (5ft 4in), you'll probably want a 55cm ball. If you're 1.65m (5ft 5in) to 1.8m (5ft 11in), go with 65cm. Taller people should look for a 75cm ball. Your hips should be level with or just slightly higher than your knees when you sit on it. The staff at your local sports shop can advise you on your individual needs.

of a painting or photograph, and the image materialises before your eyes. Buy the biggest jigsaw you can handle – some have thousands of pieces – and devote a card table or other surface to this low-tech, stress-relieving pursuit. Listen to your favourite music as you work at it and you'll happily let the television stay dark for the evening (and, if the puzzle's big enough, many evenings to come). It's just as good a solitary activity as it is fun for the whole family.

Play a game of musical massage with your partner. For an evening with a difference, load a CD player that accepts multiple discs with romantic music (or use an MP3 player and speakers). You make half the selections and your partner makes half. Light a candle and turn out the lights. Turn on the music and be sure to set the player on random or 'shuffle' mode. The rules of the game are simple. When a song you selected is playing, you give the massage. When a song your partner selected is playing, your partner gives the massage.

Organise your family photos. Even in these digital days, what household doesn't have a pile of photographs that need to be organised? Dispensing with this source of clutter will be stress relief in itself, but you also will get an emotional lift when you see the photos again. If you don't already have a photo organisation system, find a shoebox or another box that's the right width to accommodate photographs. Use cardboard rectangles as dividers between categories of photos or buy a photo box which already has these dividers.

whip it together!

Sweet balsamic onion hummus

You and your friends have planned an impromptu card game – you need a healthy, quick snack to serve. This spread does the trick. Serve with whole-wheat crackers or crunchy veggies.

In a pan, heat 1 teaspoon of **olive oil**. Add 75g chopped **sweet onion** and sauté for 5 minutes. Add in 2 teaspoons of balsamic vinegar and continue to cook for 2 to 3 minutes. Remove pan from heat and set aside. In a blender combine the following:

1 can (410g) **chickpeas**

2 crushed **garlic** cloves

1 tablespoon finely chopped **red onion**

1 teaspoon chopped fresh **thyme**

1 teaspoon chopped fresh **oregano**

2 tablespoons fresh **lemon juice**

2 tablespoons **olive oil**

Salt and **pepper** to taste

Add the onion mixture to blender and blend again until smooth.

Exercise with your dog. If you have a large dog, you probably already get some pretty good exercise taking it for walks. But you might also like to try this indoor activity to burn a few more calories. Teach your faithful friend to tug on one end of a length of rope while you hold the other. Holding your elbow at your side, slowly raise your hand to your shoulder and lower it again (the bicep curl motion). When your bicep (the muscle on the front of your upper arm) tires, exercise the tricep (the muscle on the back): starting with your arm straight down at your side, move your hand backwards, pulling on the rope, and then return your hand to the starting position. When one arm tires, switch to the other arm and repeat both exercises.

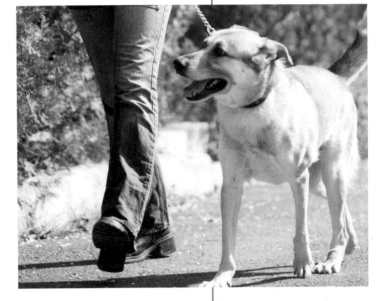

Active training for Fido. Here's another enjoyable way to get a bit of indoor action (but it's best with a well-trained pet!). Give your dog a command to stay in the kitchen, and then go and hide elsewhere in the house – behind the sofa, behind a door or in a cupboard, for instance. Then call your dog. If he obeyed the command until you called and was able to find you, give him a treat. A few rounds of hide-and-seek will reinforce your pet's training and give you a bit of exercise as well.

Offer 15 minutes of 'fetch'. For this activity, you need a large room – at least 3m long or more. Stand at one end of this 'runway' and toss a toy or ball for your dog. Choose an item that won't harm the floor, walls or furniture – preferably one that makes a noise. Dogs love this kind of game and most will return the ball to you again and again. Every time you receive the ball, do a knee-bend as you take it from the dog's mouth. Your dog may be doing more work, but the throwing, bending and reaching is doing you some good as well.

Play 'fish' with the cat. Go to the petshop and buy a 'cat-fishing' toy – a long plastic rod with a string on one end that dangles a feathery toy. When you get home, stand in the living room holding the rod and letting the toy rest against the floor. Your cat will creep towards the toy. Test your own reflexes against your cat's: can you snatch the toy away just before she pounces? You and your cat will have fun and exercise with this classic cat toy.

Burn calories at home

You know that exercise is a fundamental part of managing diabetes, but excuses to avoid it are more plentiful than daffodils in the spring. It's too rainy to go for a walk. It's too cold. The shopping centre, with its sheltered walkways, is too full of teenagers. With some basic home equipment, the living room can be your own private gym. (Or put the equipment in the spare room or basement.) And, of course, household chores can also provide a vigorous workout.

Vow to keep clothes and junk from cluttering the treadmill. A treadmill is exercise equipment, but if you treat it like a clothes rack or an extra shelf, you're hardly likely to use it – so don't clutter it up in the first place! When your exercise equipment is at the ready for a workout, you have one less excuse standing between you and your health goals.

Jump on your bike or treadmill before 10am. Researchers say that people who do their workouts early are more likely to stick to their exercise plans because the task is completed before other tasks distract you. There's an added health bonus, too: exercise produces feel-good brain chemicals called endorphins, which will give you a lift that will last the better part of the day.

Move your feet to a high-energy beat. Before you jump on your treadmill or stationary bike, turn on some high-energy music. Scientists say people exercise 5 to 15 per cent harder when they're listening to upbeat tunes.

PLUS POINT
Scientists say upbeat music makes exercisers work harder.

Listen to a good book while working out. Web sites for large book retailers, such as Amazon.co.uk, sell audio CDs of contemporary novels (libraries have them, too). Pop your purchase into your disc player, raise your right hand, and make a promise to yourself: 'No matter how engaging I find this story to be, I will only listen to this recorded book while I am walking on the treadmill in the sitting room'. You'll find yourself actually looking forward to your workout – it's the only way to find out what happens in the next chapter.

Make a weekly or twice-weekly date with your vacuum cleaner. Not only will this help ensure that your feet are protected from debris, but vacuuming also burns nearly 240kcal an hour. And your flooring – whether it's carpeting, wood, tile or vinyl – will last longer and look nicer if it's kept free of abrasive, ground-in dirt.

Make your living room an oasis

Stress and high blood glucose go hand in hand. Instead of seeking food or mindless television to relieve your tension and anxiety, try one of the soothing approaches outlined below. Making even one small change in your daily routine can add up to a calmer outlook and feeling that you are more in control of your life.

Compose a heartfelt letter on pretty stationery. In an era of mobile phones, emails and instant messaging, penning a letter and hand-addressing the envelope is a gratifying return to simpler ways, not to mention a wonderful way to keep in touch with those you love. And what a treat it will be when the return letters start outnumbering the junk mail and bills that arrive through your letterbox. Get started by keeping these items in the drawer of your coffee table or desk: a comfortable fountain pen that you love to write with, stationery that's appropriate for all occasions, your address book and stamps.

Make afternoon tea a daily ritual. Teatime is relaxing, and being relaxed can prevent stress hormones from raising your blood

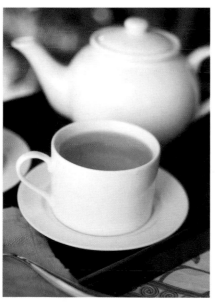

glucose. Did you know that both the black and green varieties of tea help protect your vascular system? In one study, people who were heavy tea drinkers were 44 per cent less likely to die after they had a heart attack than people who did not consume tea. And tea consumption appears to help prevent health problems in the first place – including heart attacks and diabetes. Scientists believe that tea

>> continued on page 76

---

golden rule

Keep your shoes on

Your living room may have wall-to-wall carpet, but that doesn't mean you should stroll around barefoot. Protecting your feet is important for people with diabetes, particularly if the condition has left you with reduced feeling in your feet, which makes it more difficult for you to tell if your feet are injured. Even on that plush carpet, it's still possible to step on sharp objects or stub a toe. If you have hard flooring in your living areas, wear shoes or slippers that provide cushioning under your feet and support around the ankles. This rule applies when you are on holiday, too.

Meditation

When you hear the word 'meditation', a slight frown probably crosses your face. Isn't meditation a 'fringe' activity for hippie-types who like to burn incense? In short, no. It's simply a way to distract your mind for a few minutes from your churning thoughts and your daily worries – no incense or 'lotus' positions required. And you can do it from your easy chair.

For a person who has diabetes, there are very real physical benefits to meditating – especially if you're feeling stressed, anxious or out-of-control. It can help you to calm your mind and body, reducing your levels of stress hormones. This in turn can lower your blood pressure and boost your immune-system activity (helpful because, in people with diabetes, wounds can take longer to heal). Daily meditation can even reduce the risk of heart attack and stroke.

Meditation isn't a way to escape your life; it's a way to let yourself feel more comfortable with it – and who doesn't want that? Follow these tips to get started.

1 Easy steps to get ready

Wear comfortable clothes. Put on loose clothing that does not pull, squeeze or restrict you. Make sure that your belt and shoes are not too tight or causing you discomfort.

Pick just the right spot. Comfort is key. So is serenity – be sure to choose a quiet spot where you'll be free from noise and other external distractions. The easy chair in your living room is a fine candidate if you're not too slumped in it – a straighter posture may promote mental alertness and lessen your chances of falling asleep. It also allows for freer, easier breathing. Some people prefer sitting on the floor, perhaps near an open window.

Have a clear view of the clock. You will want to know when your meditation time is over, so position a clock within sight of your meditating spot. Your watch won't do because you don't want to have to lift your arm and focus on the small numbers to read the time.

Choose a word. Call it a mantra if you wish, but really it's just one calming word (preferably just one or two syllables) that you can focus on while you meditate. Words like 'peace' and 'joy' are good candidates. Another school of thought is to pick a sound like 'om' so that you're focusing on your breathing rather than the meaning of the word.

2 Focus on two simple things

Once you're ready, distract your mind for 10 to 15 minutes. You may close your eyes or leave them open – it's up to you. If you prefer your eyes closed, you will need to open them occasionally so you will know when your 15 minutes have passed. Focus on just two things: your breathing and your word or sound.

Breathe deeply and pay attention to the air as it enters and leaves your lungs. It doesn't matter whether you breathe through your mouth or your nose.

Repeat your chosen word or sound to yourself in your head each time you exhale. If any other thought starts creeping into your head, consciously direct your mind back to your word or sound and to your breathing. Keep everything else outside the bubble of peace that you're in. When your breathing becomes completely relaxed, you won't even hear yourself inhale or exhale. Your goal is to be awake and alert, but not at all tense.

3 Time's up – now what?

Meditation feels better and better over time. Try doing it every day. Don't give up: it could easily take eight weeks for you to be completely comfortable meditating. Eventually, you'll learn to stop 'talking to yourself' in your head, which can be difficult. And you'll slip into a state of alert relaxation faster and faster. Once you have the hang of it and meditation feels natural, do it three times per week, 15 minutes per session. But start off with small sessions, since even a few minutes meditation is better than none.

Besides helping you manage your diabetes, meditating regularly can make you a calmer, more efficient person, and it should improve your interactions with others.

4 Guided imagery: another way to relax

Think of guided imagery as a wonderful holiday without the hassle of security checks and baggage reclaim. Led by a voice on an audiotape or CD, you relax while the person leads you through a series of comfortable mental experiences involving all of the senses, beautiful vistas and welcoming people. Your body responds as if what you're imagining is real. Tapes are designed for specific purposes, such as reducing stress, managing pain, losing weight and easing insomnia. Look for them wherever you buy music or books on tape.

A related practice, called visualisation, requires no tapes, just your imagination. Here you picture a relaxing scene using all your senses. For instance, try to imagine yourself relaxing on a sunny beach. See the seagulls diving for fish, feel the wind on your face and the sand beneath your feet, smell the air, listen to the crash of the waves. Close your eyes and feel you're there. You may even be able to taste the tang of salty water from the ocean spray.

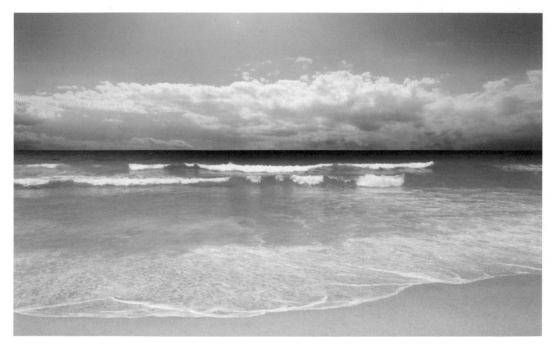

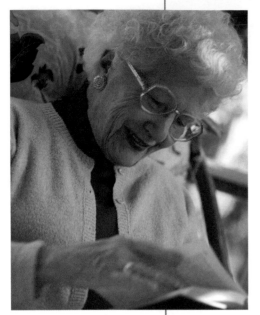

keeps your blood vessels supple, helps to prevent artery blockages and discourages blood clots. And, if you really cannot drink your tea unsweetened, use an artificial sweetener.

Get a chair that rocks. Buy a rocking chair for your living room and sit in it, saving the recliner for a guest. During one of your favourite films or TV programmes keep the rocking chair going. That level of activity may seem minimal, but every little bit helps. And over the course of an evening, all that rocking adds up to a fair amount of foot and calf stretching, and much more than if you'd been slumped on a settee.

Turn some pages for motivation. Reading is relaxing – and it can also be motivating. How many of those books by your easy chair contain some element of health, sports or physical activity? If your answer is 'none', visit the library and ask for recommendations that will put you in an active, healthy mindset. Try the autobiographies of Kelly Holmes or Steve Redgrave for inspiration. Or look at a travel guide and plan an active holiday. And try to find inspiring tales of individuals who have overcome major obstacles; they will make the ones you face seem infinitely small and highly manageable.

Don't draw the curtains if it's still light outside. Natural light boosts your levels of the feel-good brain chemical serotonin. Not much sun outside your window? You can now buy light bulbs that simulate natural sunshine; their blue wavelength, which is missing in conventional light bulbs, makes all the difference.

Put noises on 'mute'. Blaring, jarring noises make your living space more stressful. Buy headphones for use with your television, computer and audio systems so that their users won't fill the house with unwanted sound. Carpet your living room if possible, and favour upholstered furniture. If you and your partner use noisy appliances frequently, strike an agreement with him or her to establish some quiet hours each evening. If noise from the outside is a real problem, consider installing noise-reducing windows.

Warm up your living space with autumnal colours. Decorating your home in warm yellow, gold, orange and red tones will warm up your mood, too. Rehabilitation facilities use this golden colour scheme to keep patients upbeat and happy – and it's no surprise that it works, because it mimics the effect of sunlight.

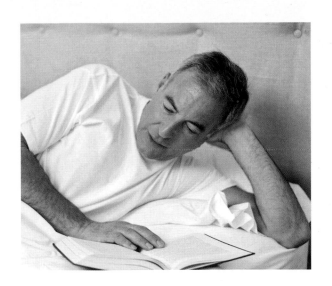

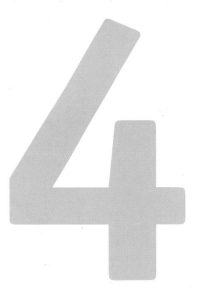

In your bedroom

The bedroom brings its own set of

pleasures, from luxurious sleep –

important for good blood glucose

control – to relaxing reading or stress-

relieving private time with your

partner. Make your bedroom a

haven for body and soul.

Getting quality sleep

Long-term lack of sleep can make blood glucose levels harder to manage by reducing your body's sensitivity to insulin, the hormone that moves glucose out of the bloodstream and into your cells. It can also boost the risk of a long list of medical problems, including obesity, high blood pressure, heart attacks and strokes. If you don't feel well rested when you wake in the morning, take steps to address the problem. The payoff of deep, luxurious slumber is worth the effort.

golden rule

Get at least 8 hours of sleep every night

Can poor sleep lead to poor blood glucose control? Perhaps. Researchers at the University of Chicago studied 161 people who have Type 2 diabetes. Only 6 per cent of the patients were getting 8 hours' sleep a night, and 70 per cent of them reported routinely getting poor-quality sleep. Lack of sleep or poor quality of sleep were closely associated with higher HbA1c scores, a measure of blood glucose levels over the long term. 'We've known for some time that skimping on sleep can impair glucose tolerance for healthy people,' said researcher Kristen Knutson. 'Now we have evidence connecting chronic partial sleep deprivation and reduced blood-sugar control in patients with diabetes.'

Go to bed and wake up at a similar time every day. Your body likes routines, so give it a dependable sleep schedule. Try to go to bed at about the same time every night and wake at around the same time every morning, even on weekends. You'll fall asleep faster, and be more likely to get the right amount of sleep.

If you do want a lie in, do a quick blood glucose test. Controlling your blood glucose and lying in on your day off can seem downright incompatible for people who are on insulin. But with a little effort, you can do both. Here's an example, the night before the day you want a lie in, set the alarm for a relatively early time – say, 6am. When the alarm goes off, check your blood glucose. If it's high or normal, you will need a couple of units of soluble (rapid or quick acting) insulin because your blood glucose will be rising. If your blood glucose is low, drink a glass of juice or milk. Then jump back into bed and close your eyes for a few more hours, secure in the knowledge that your blood glucose is under control. If you don't feel confident about doing this without medical advice, discuss the timing and dosages with a health professional.

Aim to get at least 30 minutes of exercise a day, five times a week. Physical activity is a boon to so many body functions, and sleep is one of them. The gentle fatigue that you get from exercise will set your body up for a good night's rest. So for the sake of shut-eye – on top of all of the other health benefits – stick to your physical activity plans.

Wind down 3 hours before bedtime. Wind down in the evening, reducing your activity level as bedtime approaches. Start relaxing 3 hours before lights-out. One hour before you go to bed, do something quiet and peaceful – take a bath, stretch gently, read or listen to pleasant music. Twenty minutes before bedtime, dim the lights. By the time you pull your covers up under your chin, your eyelids should be drooping.

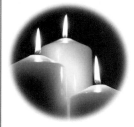

Check your blood glucose regularly. Either high or low blood glucose levels can affect your sleep. If you're not feeling fully rested in the morning, being aware of how your blood glucose levels vary during the day and night will help you to take steps to keep your blood glucose steady.

PLUS POINT
Regulating your blood glucose will help you to avoid the highs and lows that can affect your sleep.

If you are having trouble sleeping, check your blood glucose. Set your alarm for 3am every morning for one week and check your blood glucose each time. If you find consistently normal readings, that should set your mind at rest. If you find that your blood glucose is below 4mmol/l when you check it at 3am, eat a snack. Keep a high carbohydrate snack in the drawer of your bedside table for this purpose, and have a bottle of water handy to wash it down. If you discover that your blood glucose is consistently low in the middle of the night, talk to your health professional about the possibility of adjusting your nighttime insulin dose or the snack you eat (if any) before going to bed.

Nod off in total darkness. Draw the curtains so that they block out as much light as possible. Even better, buy blackout curtains or blinds that are specially designed to block out sunlight. In addition, make sure that there are no glowing electronic devices in your bedroom, such as televisions, alarm clocks or nightlights that might distract you from sleep. And be sure to switch off your mobile phone.

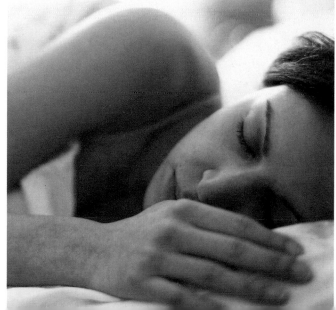

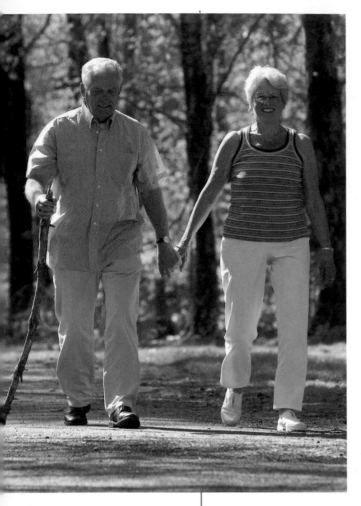

Keep a torch by the bed. When you wake during the night needing a trip to the bathroom, you don't want to wake your partner by turning on the light. But stumbling around in the dark just invites a stubbed toe. A torch directed at the floor just in front of you will escort you safely to the bathroom and back.

Let nocturnal noises fall on deaf ears. Trying to sleep in a noisy setting is difficult, and it may even raise your blood pressure. So it's worth investing a little time and money to make your bedroom as quiet as possible. If your partner watches the evening news in bed while you're trying to nod off, buy him or her a set of cordless headphones. If his or her snoring keeps you awake, invest in some earplugs. To block out street noise, you could pop in a CD that plays nature sounds or buy a 'white noise' machine, which generates a dull yet calming sound that covers other noises. In summer turn on a fan and let its whirr lull you to sleep.

Turn down the thermostat. Researchers at the University of South Australia have found that insomniacs have a higher core body temperature than those who don't have trouble sleeping. The university's Centre for Sleep Research experts say that the body starts to lose heat between 60 and 90 minutes before you fall asleep. If you're not sleeping well, you can help your body wind down by keeping your bedroom moderately cool – say, between 20°C and 22°C, or cooler if you prefer.

If you've had a beer, have a healthy snack, too. If you've enjoyed a glass of wine or beer in the hours leading up to your bedtime, do a quick check of your glucose levels. If your blood glucose is low, have a small snack if you need one before getting under the covers. Alcohol makes it more difficult for your body to recover from low blood glucose; a bite to eat will moderate its effects.

Stop drinking a short time before bedtime. To reduce your nocturnal urination, and therefore interrupted sleep, avoid diuretics such as tea and coffee in the evening, and don't drink liquids of any kind in the 2 hours before you go to bed. If you put less fluid in the 'pipeline' before you hit the sack, there will be less fluid building up in your bladder during the night.

If you have chronic pain, invest in a high-quality mattress. These mattresses may cost more, but are worth it. Even buying a firm conventional mattress could help you to sleep better.

Use a thin pillow if you sleep on your back. A plump pillow could compromise your body alignment and cause pain in your neck, if you sleep on your back. However, if you prefer to sleep on your side, a well-stuffed pillow will provide better neck support and therefore better sleep.

Test yourself for sleep apnoea. Does your partner say you snore loudly or seem to be holding your breath while you sleep? You might have sleep apnoea, a malady that interrupts the rhythmic breathing that other sleepers enjoy. Sleep apnoea can aggravate diabetes-related conditions such as high blood pressure, obesity and impotence. It also raises the risk of heart disease. If you sleep alone and always wake up exhausted, set up a noise-activated recorder before you go to bed to help you rule out sleep apnoea. If you suspect you have it, discuss your concerns with your doctor, who can refer you for further tests.

Let yourself see the sunshine. According to research, sunlight is a powerful regulator of hormones that control sleeping and waking. When it's exposed to sunlight, your body knows to inhibit production of the sleep-inducing hormone melatonin, and when night falls, melatonin goes into high production. If you're housebound and not sleeping well, lack of sun exposure could be the reason.

Make your bedtime drink a decaf – or a cup of herbal tea. Reducing or eliminating your caffeine intake will go a long way in helping you to get a better night's sleep. Check the labels for the caffeine content of your soft drinks and herbal tea – some herbal teas do contain caffeine. Try to avoid having anything containing caffeine for 6 hours before you go to bed.

Avoid naps or limit them. If you're napping during the day and not sleeping well at night, you might be napping too much. The

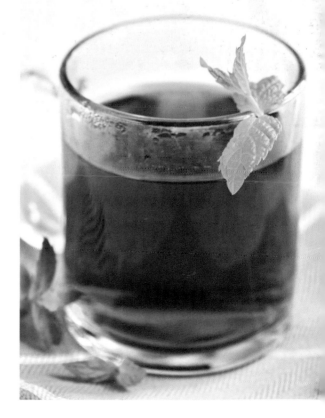

British Medical Journal recommends avoiding naps if you suffer from insomnia. Other medical experts suggest no more than 20-30 minutes daytime napping and a deadline – finish your nap by 3pm.

Talk to your doctor if you're feeling low. Research shows that people with diabetes are at a greater risk of depression than people who do not have diabetes, although the reasons for this are unknown. Depression can interfere with sleep. If you find yourself lying awake early in the morning and feeling hopeless or 'down', talk about it with your GP. It's possible that treatment for depression, which may include medication, counselling, or both, will put you on the path to better sleep. Simply acknowledging you feel low or depressed can be helpful in itself.

Write down your to-do list before you go to sleep. How many times do we lie down and drift off only to jolt awake because we have forgotten to pay a bill or make an appointment? Keep a notebook

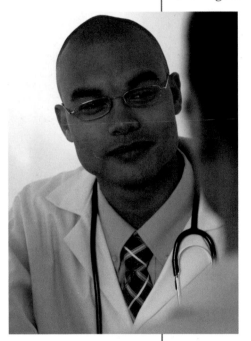

by the bed so that you can write down things that you have to do the next day, or any other worries that have been nagging you throughout the day, to free your mind for sleep.

Tell your doctor if you experience a stinging pain in your legs. If a painful sensation that feels a little like bees attacking your feet is keeping you awake at night, ask your doctor to consider whether you might have neuropathy (nerve damage) in your legs. Treatments for another condition, restless leg syndrome, are frequently advertised, but don't assume that's the problem – neuropathy is different. Prescription drugs including certain antidepressants and anticonvulsants can provide relief for this sleep-robbing malady, or your doctor may be able to recommend over-the-counter painkillers such as aspirin or ibuprofen. Some people find that walking regularly or wearing elastic stockings helps, too.

Rub on pepper cream to relieve foot pain. Creams that contain capsaicin, the 'hot' ingredient in hot peppers, may provide relief for people who have foot pain caused by nerve damage, and they can be prescribed for you. Rub some onto your feet three or four times a day. Initially, the cream will provide a warm sensation. Over several weeks, the nerve pain will subside. Be sure to wash your hands immediately after applying the cream, or use protective gloves to apply it, and make sure it doesn't come in contact with your face.

Creating a stress-free oasis

You spend about a third of your life in the bedroom, so why not make it a comfortable, soothing refuge? Remember, reducing stress helps reduce high blood glucose, since stress blocks the release of insulin. Here are a few tips to help you transform your bedroom's atmosphere.

Clear your room of clutter. Smooth, clean surfaces act as a balm on your brain, so clear away clutter, put away all the clothes strewn on your bedroom chair, and buy a bookshelf for that stack of books collecting dust.

Once a week, put fresh flowers in your room. An American study found that female office workers felt more relaxed when they were working near a vase of flowers. Just imagine how nice it would feel to sleep near one.

Scent your room with essential oils. In aromatherapy, a number of scents are recognised as particularly useful for reducing stress. There are several easy ways to introduce these scents into your bedroom. One is to buy a light bulb ring (a device that you set onto a cold light bulb), add a couple of drops of essential oil, and turn on the lamp to let the oil warm and scent the air. Another is to buy or make potpourri, a collection of dried herbs treated with essential oils. Or mix in a spray bottle 50ml of water, plus a drop or two of your favourite oils, and use the scent as an air freshener. Relaxing scents include bergamot, chamomile, lavender, lemon, marjoram, neroli, orange, sandalwood, valerian and ylang ylang.

When choosing bedroom hues, go for blue. Scientists say that the colour blue affects the autonomic nervous system – the part that operates without your conscious control – to lower the heart rate and blood pressure, and slow the breathing. Proponents of colour therapy say that blue has a calming, relaxing effect and helps lull you to sleep. If the room is due for a fresh coat of paint, go for a blue tone. If not, try adding sky-coloured blankets, pillows and rugs.

Try a few feng shui tips. Feng shui aims to achieve harmony between your spiritual self and your physical environment. According to this ancient discipline, proper positioning of elements of a room creates the desired energy flow and balance of forces. Practitioners recommend that you position your bed on the opposite side of the room from the bedroom door – not directly in front of the door, but diagonally across the room from it; position the bed so that when you lie in it, a window is to your right (to feed you positive energy when you wake up); and keep desks and computers, along with their work-related energy, out of the bedroom.

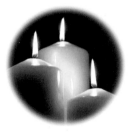

PLUS POINT

Go for blue. Colour therapists say blue hues have the most calming and relaxing effects.

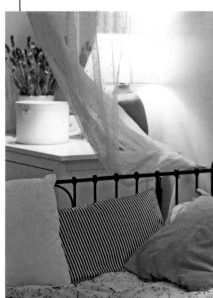

Diabetes and your sex life

Making love with your partner is a wonderful activity for your relationship and for your health. And people who have diabetes can enjoy fully satisfying sex lives. Like most things with diabetes, some thinking ahead might be needed to make your romantic encounters more successful and enjoyable.

Use exercise to increase your libido. Here's yet further motivation to get your recommended daily dose of physical activity: both men and women with diminished sex drive benefit from regular aerobic exercise, experts say. Exercise improves your blood flow, which will improve the function and sensitivity of your sex organs. Stronger muscles, better aerobic capacity and an improved self-image will also enhance your experience in the bedroom.

Check your blood glucose before making love. If your blood glucose tends to drop during physical activity or at night, having sex can present a challenge. Before things get too heated, check your blood glucose so that you're sure of your status. If your blood glucose is at the normal level or is already on the low side, you may need to adjust your insulin or eat something before or after sex – a robust session could make you hypoglycaemic. If you have an insulin pump, consider unhooking it during sex.

Be careful if you're making love after you have had a drink. Alcohol and vigorous sex both lower blood glucose, and combining the two could cause a dangerous low. Make sure that you monitor your blood glucose if drinking alcohol is going to be part of your romantic evening.

If your libido is flagging, ask yourself two questions. First: does your reduced sexual desire apply to all situations at all times? If so, review with your doctor the possible medical sources of your diminished sex drive. Medications you're taking or hormone problems could be the culprit. If the answer to the first question is 'no', ask yourself: does the strength of your sex drive depend on the situation? Perhaps you have little desire for sex with your partner, but you find other people attractive and get satisfaction from masturbation. If so, marital or couples counselling could help.

Massage your partner tonight, and get a return massage tomorrow night. The added relaxation may help to reduce your levels of stress hormones, which can drive up your blood glucose. This kind of touch is a nice way to connect with your spouse and show you care. A bonus for the massage giver: because massaging someone takes force, your hands and arms get some exercise.

PLUS POINT
Sex can act like insulin, lowering your blood glucose.

golden rule

Discuss sexual problems with your GP

Set bashfulness aside, and tell your doctor if your sex drive is significantly lower than it used to be. Hiding the problem can weigh on your mind, leading to self-blame and despair, making your sexual performance even worse. For a person with diabetes, a number of factors could be responsible for reduced sex drive. Your doctor will know how to identify potential causes and get you the appropriate care.

Be especially touchy if you or your partner has nerve damage. It's rare, but in some cases nerve damage reduces sensitivity in the genitals in people who have diabetes. In some cases you can compensate for this with additional gentle touching in the right places.

Report cloudy urine or pain during intercourse to your GP. High blood glucose compromises the body's ability to fend off bacterial infection. If you feel pain during sex (especially for women), have urine that's clouded or bloody, get a burning sensation when you urinate, or constantly feel the need to urinate, talk to your doctor. You may have a urinary tract infection. Refrain from sex until the problem is resolved.

Don't be afraid to use lubricants. Among women who have diabetes, vaginal dryness is common, and it is a simple problem to remedy. Keep water-based lubricants in the drawer of your bedside table, each of them a different colour, scent or flavour. Some lubricants warm when they make contact with skin. The variety will add a degree of sensuous play to your love life, which can be a bonus if you or your partner has a flagging sex drive. Stick to water-based lubricants. Oil-based lubricants (such as petroleum jelly) can damage condoms and lead to bacterial infections.

Prevent surprise pregnancies. Apart from the obvious stress involved with an unplanned pregnancy, there are additional problems for a woman who has diabetes. If you're pregnant and your blood glucose isn't under control, you run a high risk of birth defects or a miscarriage. Your birth control options are the same as for people who do not have diabetes. However, if you use birth control pills, monitor your blood glucose closely, and ask your doctor whether you need to adjust your insulin or other medications. Birth control pills work by giving you hormones, and some hormones can raise blood glucose levels. And remember that women who have entered peri-menopause and are having irregular periods can still become pregnant.

Discuss your options for birth-control methods with your GP. There are many types of contraceptives available and the right one for you will depend on your age, lifestyle and general health as well as your diabetes and its control.

Guard against fungal infections. Women who have diabetes are more susceptible to vaginal infections and should take special care to avoid them. Higher glucose levels in the vaginal lining, combined with moisture and warmth, encourage the growth of bacteria and yeast. The problem is particularly bad for older women because levels of protective oestrogen drop around menopause. Bathe regularly and keep the vaginal area dry, and avoid clothing that will hold moisture against you. Avoid harsh feminine products that invite infection, including douches, feminine sprays and strong soaps. Ask your doctor about medicated ointments and creams that will clear up the problem.

To prevent bladder infection, urinate before and after sex. If you're a woman with damage to the nerves controlling your bladder (neurogenic bladder), try to urinate just before sex and within 30 minutes afterwards to reduce your chance of developing an infection.

Don't be too embarrassed to talk to your GP. Impotence is sometimes an issue for people with diabetes. A wide range of factors – for instance, nerve damage and blood flow problems – can contribute

Is your menstrual cycle affecting your blood glucose?

Your menstrual cycle might be complicating your efforts to manage your diabetes. Women build up high levels of oestrogen and progesterone about a week before menstruation. Some scientists believe that these hormones interfere with insulin sensitivity in many women, most often making blood glucose run high, but sometimes causing it to drop. So take out your record of blood glucose readings for the last three months and mark the dates when your last three periods began. Were your blood glucose levels high a week before each period? If so, experiment with some ways to avoid this: exercising a bit more around this time might help, for example. If you use insulin and you are used to altering your dose, increasing your dose by a unit or two and reducing it again when your period starts, might help. If your blood glucose tends to drop a week before your period, the reverse action might work, for example temporarily eating a bit more and lowering your insulin dose slightly.

to erection problems, as can some of the blood-pressure medications taken by many diabetics. A large number of men who have diabetes and are over the age of 50 encounter erection problems. Your doctor won't be surprised to hear about your condition and can help you.

Identify the underlying cause of your impotence. Some doctors are quick to write a prescription without taking a medical history and looking for underlying medical problems. Don't settle for an erection stimulating pill as your first and only answer. By identifying what is causing the problem, you can find the best solution for you.

Take ginkgo biloba to give your blood flow a boost. This herbal supplement is said to improve blood flow. Since an erection is basically a matter of hydraulics – blood flowing to the penis – taking gingko regularly could lead to better erections. Check with your doctor

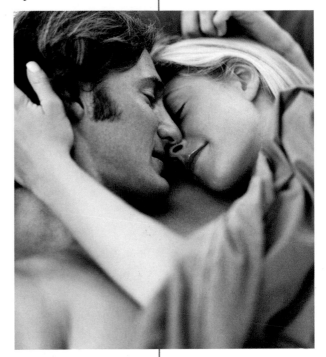

before taking this supplement, however, because it can interact with other medications.

Test yourself for night-time erections. Erectile dysfunction problems can be physical or emotional. Here's an easy way to tell the difference. Before bedtime, wrap a small strip of paper around your penis and tape the ends together to form a band (don't put tape all the way around the penis). If the paper is broken in the morning, you probably had an erection.

If a man is having erection problems during sex because of emotional issues, he will probably still have erections while he sleeps. The more scientific way to detect nocturnal erections is to be monitored during sleep, either in a sleep lab or with a monitor you use in your own bed. If you are not having erections during sleep, your problems are more likely to be physical.

Get a prostate check up. If your sleep is frequently interrupted by trips to the bathroom, ask your doctor whether your prostate could be causing the problem. If your prostate is enlarged, it could be squeezing the urethra, the tube that urine passes through on its way out of the body. The result of that squeezing is that you feel as if you need to urinate more often.

Treat your feet to TLC

Everyone gets a blister or callus now and then, but these can be much more serious for you if you have poor circulation or reduced feeling in your feet. Poor blood circulation makes healing more difficult and because of nerve damage, you might not feel sores, blisters or cuts. Foot problems left untreated could even lead to amputation. So make examining your feet every night a bedtime ritual.

Get your partner to play 'footsie' with you. There are many reasons you might find it difficult to check your feet thoroughly: back problems, obesity and arthritis may reduce the flexibility you need to inspect your feet closely. Diminished eyesight makes the task harder, too. In any case, enlist your partner's help. The slight inconvenience that it might be to ask for someone's help is a lot better than finding out about foot injuries too late.

Keep a small mirror under your bed. It's pretty easy to see the tops and sides of your feet, but many people aren't agile enough to get a good look at the bottoms. If you have this quandary, buy a shatter-proof mirror that's about the size of a sheet of notebook paper and place it mirror-side up under your bed. At bedtime, use your toes to slide the mirror out from under the bed. Examine your feet in the mirror, and then slide the mirror back into its hiding place.

Keep your eyes open for irritations large and small. When you conduct your foot check, you obviously need to keep an eye out for open sores and cuts. Signs of infection in a sore include swelling, redness, drainage, oozing or excess warmth. Contact a health professional promptly if you see any of these symptoms around a sore, at the site of a splinter or cut, or around your toenails. Smaller signs of irritation need quick attention, too, including redness, corns or calluses. Pay particular attention to the toes and the ball of your foot – that's where most foot ulcers develop.

Clean and treat minor scrapes and cuts right away. Wash your hands with soap and water. Then wash the wound with soap and water, rinse with more water, and pat it dry with a clean towel or paper towel. Taking a little antibiotic ointment on a cotton

golden rule

Examine your feet every night when you go to bed

When you get into your car, you buckle your seatbelt without thinking. Make examining your feet just as automatic. Every night when you pull off your shoes and socks, add one more step to your undressing routine: a thorough check-up for your feet. Start with your toes, then do the bottoms, sides, tops and ankles. Regularity is the key. You never know when a foot problem might surface, and catching it early will help you to avoid serious complications, including ulcers, severe infections and even amputation.

make the change

The habit: Working with your health-care team to establish a foot-care programme.

The result: Reducing your risk of amputation by half.

The evidence: Several large medical centres have established comprehensive foot-care programmes for people who have diabetes. These include treatment for foot problems, preventive therapy, patient education, referral to specialists and referral to shoe fitters. With such programmes, centres have found that they can reduce the amputations they perform by 45 to 85 per cent. Ask your doctor or podiatrist if there's a programme at a hospital near you.

swab, smear a thin layer onto the wound. (Don't apply the ointment with your finger.) Cover the wound with a plaster or padded bandage. If the wound does not look better within a day, or if you see signs of infection, such as swelling, redness, excess warmth or oozing, contact a health professional promptly. If you are not sure which cream is suitable for you, ask your podiatrist or a health professional.

Moisturise your feet. When you take your socks off, check to see if tiny white flakes – dry skin cells – fall to the floor. If you see them, your skin is too dry, and you'll need to moisturise with a thick cream or lotion. If you don't moisturise, your skin could begin to crack, leaving you vulnerable to infection. Pay particular attention to your heels and the balls of your feet, where dryness is most likely. Then tuck your feet into clean cotton socks, which not only keep your sheets from being streaked with lotion, they also seal the moisture into your skin. Applying moisturiser once or twice a day should be enough to keep skin from cracking.

Ask your podiatrist to trim your toenails. Health-care professionals are sometimes reluctant to let you care for

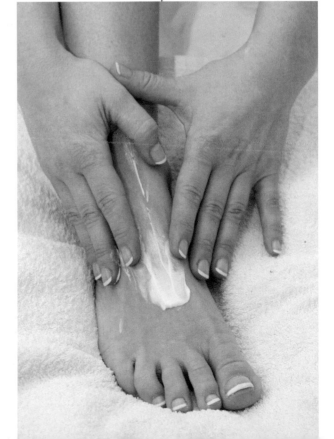

>> continued on page 92

Exercise in bed!

It's no fun getting out of bed only to be greeted by a chorus of complaining joints. Here's a set of gentle stretches and muscle-toning exercises you can do while you're still lying in bed. They should help to reduce your stiffness and put you in the mood for the kind of physically active day that will help you to control your diabetes. Start with just a few repetitions of each exercise and build up to the recommended number.

1 Knee pull

Lie on your back. **Raise** your left knee and wrap both hands around the front of it. Gently **pull** your knee towards your chest and then **return** to the starting position. Repeat two to four more times. Then change sides. This will stretch your lower back and the backs of your legs.

2 Front stretch

Lie face down with your palms on the bed near your shoulders. Keeping your hips against the bed, **push** down to raise your head and chest. **Exhale** as you push, and stop when your elbows form a right angle. Hold for 5 to 10 seconds. Exhale as you **lower** yourself to the starting position. Repeat three to five more times. This will stretch the muscles in your abdomen, chest, and lower back.

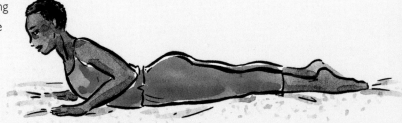

3 Thigh and groin stretch

Lie on your left side. **Move** your right leg behind you and **reach** back with your right hand to grasp the top of your right foot just behind your toes, or ankle. **Arch** your back slightly and hold for 5 to 10 seconds. Repeat two to four more times. Switch to lying on your right side and repeat. This will stretch the tops of your thighs and the groin.

4 Tummy tightener

Lie on your back with your knees bent and your feet flat on the bed. **Lean** your head forward slightly and **reach** until your fingers touch your knees. Hold for 5 seconds, and **return** to the starting position. Repeat nine more times. This exercise strengthens your stomach muscles.

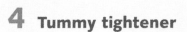

5 Foot push

Lie on your back in bed with your feet flat against the footboard (or turn around and place your feet against the headboard). **Press** against the board with your toes, hold for 5 seconds, and **release**. Repeat nine more times. This exercise strengthens your calf muscles and ankles.

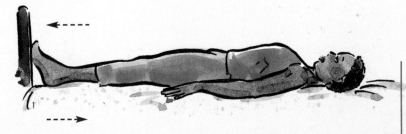

your own toenails if you have nerve damage or poor circulation, or if you struggle to reach your toes, because sharp clippers can cause accidental injuries. Be honest: can you reach your toes easily? Do you have a good set of toenail clippers? Will you take the time to trim them meticulously? If the answer is 'no', ask someone else to do the task for you, or better yet, ask your podiatrist to do it.

If you do trim your own nails, use clippers designed for toenails. Toenail clippers are larger and have more leverage than fingernail clippers, so they can snip through thicker toenails without you having to apply excess pressure, which could lead to injury. Also, their blades are less rounded, which makes them more suitable for bigger toes. You can purchase lever-style toenail clippers (which look like oversized fingernail clippers) or scissor-style clippers (which look like mini-wire cutters) from larger pharmacies. Or you might want to use emery boards instead. To avoid unnecessary injuries, don't try to use conventional scissors, a knife or any other metal instruments, and don't tear or pull at your toenails.

Soften sharp toenail edges. When you trim your toenails, cut them so that they're flush with the tip of your toe, and slightly curved to follow the shape of your toe. You often see advice suggesting that you should clip toenails straight across, but this can leave sharp points on the sides that can cut into your skin or become ingrown. Use a file or emery board to smooth any sharp edges.

Toss out your electric blanket. Don't bed down with any devices that will create extreme temperatures, such as electric blankets, heating pads, hot water bottles and ice packs. If you have reduced feeling in your feet, you might not be able to tell when such items are overheating or over-chilling your feet or other body parts.

Slip into your slippers. A sturdy pair of nonslip slippers will protect your feet and prevent falls. Walking around barefoot is never a good idea for people with diabetes. Even if you are meticulous about housekeeping and won't risk stepping on something sharp, there are still plenty of ways in which you can stub your toe.

Check your shoes for lumps and debris. Before you put on a pair of shoes, shake them out and run your hand inside to detect pebbles, other objects, lumps, or rough linings that could rub or injure your feet. Otherwise, if you have reduced feeling in your feet, you might not notice such a problem until it's caused serious damage. Inspect the soles for any sharp pins you might have picked up, and make sure the soles are in good repair so that your feet are properly supported.

In the bathroom

You can practise better diabetes management even in the bathroom. Decisions as seemingly minor as what kind of soap to use or how hot to run your bathwater could be really important. Whether you're showering or treating your feet, follow these tips. Above all, vow never to do 'bathroom surgery' on your feet. Treating corns, calluses and ingrowing toenails is best left to the professionals.

Use moisturising bars of soap. Wash your feet daily in water that's warm but not hot. Avoid liquid soaps; they are more likely to leave your skin dry, which can lead to cracking and therefore can make you susceptible to infection. Also avoid exfoliating soaps, which can be too rough on your skin, and perfumed soaps, which cause skin reactions in some people.

Disconnect your insulin pump before showering. Even though pumps are water resistant, they shouldn't be put directly in the water. Use the disconnect port meant for swimming, bathing and showering. Read the manufacturer's instructions or ask a pump specialist or other pump users where to put the pump while you shower. For some pumps you can buy cases you can hang from a shower curtain hook.

Don't soak in a hot bath for more than 20 minutes. If you're going to have a relaxing spell in a hot tub, a hot bath, a sauna or a Jacuzzi, stay no more than 20 minutes and make sure the temperature

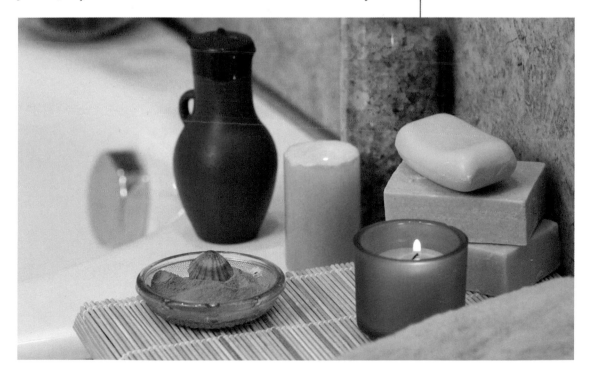

is no higher than 87°C. Excessively warm temperatures can aggravate cardiovascular problems, which are common in people with diabetes. If you're using insulin, a hot soak can increase the rate at which the body absorbs it, throwing off the timing of your blood glucose control. When you enter hot water, don't use your foot to test the temperature if you have nerve damage and loss of feeling – you might not realise that your skin is scalding. Instead, dip a hand or elbow into the water, or use a bath thermometer.

Avoid callus or corn treatments. If you have diabetes, resist the temptation to use over-the-counter treatments on the calluses and corns on your feet. When you have reduced feeling in your feet, it's easy for such treatments to damage your skin without you being aware of it. The active ingredient in both the liquids that you dab on cornsor calluses and the pads you apply is an acid that can eat away not only your dead skin, but also your healthy skin, too. The resulting wound from the acid could take a long time to heal. Don't use pumice or a file on your corns and calluses either; the risk of injury is too great, and

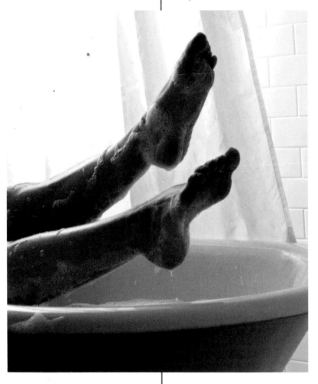

such instruments aren't sterile. Ask your doctor or podiatrist to treat any foot conditions of theis kind.

Don't use an OTC treatment for ingrowing toenails. Use of over-the-counter treatments for ingrowing toenails is also inadvisable. As with callus and corn removers, these products work by eating away the skin with acid, which puts you at risk of infection. Make an appointment with your podiatrist and have the problem treated properly.

Treat athlete's foot with medicated cream. Athlete's foot is a fungal infection which people with diabetes can safely treat with over-the-counter products. Athlete's foot appears as red, itching or cracking skin between the toes and on the bottoms of your feet. Treat this immediately, since the cracked skin can get infected. Apply athlete's foot cream twice a day. First wash your feet with soap and water. Dry them thoroughly, then rub the cream into the affected skin. Contact your GP or practice nurse if the athlete's foot hasn't cleared up within five days.

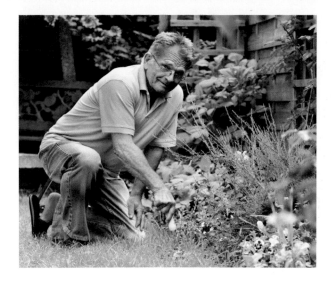

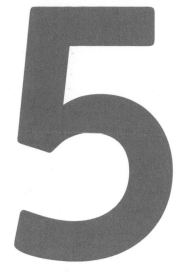

5

In your garden

Your garden is not just a place

to grow plants. It is a space where you

and your family can relax, socialise and

even cook and enjoy healthy meals.

So step outside and make

the most of outdoor living.

Good times, good friends and the great outdoors

When we speak of a home's 'living' space, we tend to talk about the floor space inside. But think about all that space in the garden. The next time friends and family pay a visit, invite everyone outside for some fun in the open air.

Invite your neighbours to a croquet party. Besides being a great theme for a fun party (if you have the space), croquet offers health benefits: you'll get a little strength training by swinging your mallet, while ambling around your garden will burn a few calories. Best of all, you'll have a few laughs and learn the latest gossip.

Keep a badminton set handy for family visits. For casual play, badminton requires little expertise and will keep everyone active and working as a team. Other easy games to keep in the garage include hula hoops, Frisbees, and ball-toss sets that use Velcro mitts.

Fit out your patio for outdoor eating. You'll need some weatherproof furniture, an umbrella or shelter of some kind and a barbecue or grill. These basics will encourage you to spend more time outdoors and serve healthy *al fresco* meals such as salads and grilled fish, chicken and lean meats.

golden rule

Vow to spend 20 minutes a day outdoors

Spending time outdoors is good for you in so many ways. Getting outside for even a few minutes a day can reduce depression. It can also help you to lose weight: light activity outside (like gardening or washing the car) burns about six times the number of calories as watching TV. And unless you live in a very northern climate, a few minutes of sunshine during months when the sun is high in the sky helps the body make vitamin D. Deficiency of this vitamin predisposes people to obesity and insulin resistance.

whip it together!

Apple coleslaw

Why drown healthy, low-calorie cabbage in fatty mayonnaise? Dressing up your coleslaw with apples, poppy seeds and low-fat condiments yields heaps of flavour with fewer calories and less fat.

In a salad bowl, combine:

1 whole shredded **green** or **red cabbage** (or a combination of both)

2 diced, unpeeled **red** or **green apples**

2 peeled and grated **carrots**

3 tablespoons **raisins**

In a separate bowl, combine:

6 tablespoons fat-free **mayonnaise**

4 tablespoons plain fat-free **yoghurt**

2 tablespoons low-fat **sour cream**

1 tablespoon **poppy seeds**

2 teaspoons apple **cider vinegar**

1 teaspoon **honey** or **sugar** substitute

Salt and **pepper** to taste

Add the dressing to the vegetable mixture and toss well. Cover and refrigerate for half an hour before serving.

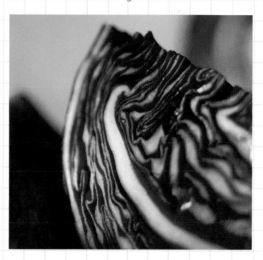

Play skipping with the little ones. Many of the old skipping games that many of us found so much fun to play at primary school, are now coming back, so a skipping rope is always a useful addition to a parent or grandparent's armoury of distractions. It's also something that can be enjoyed by one child or used for games involving a group of children – boys as well as girls. You can join in, too. Keep it in your shed or toybox and bring it out the moment the children start reaching for their headphones and electronic games. They'll be happier, fitter and more sociable as a result.

Install a bird-feeder. Watching birds is incredibly relaxing, and a feeder is what you need to bring them into your garden. Use a field guide to find out what kinds of birds you are likely to attract, and then buy a feeder and seed that suits their preferences.

Add a birdbath. Birds also need drinking and bathing water. Add four or five copper pennies to the water to prevent the formation of algae so you have to change the water less frequently.

Ready, set, grill

Lighting the barbecue or gas grill provides you with a sociable, relaxing time in the back garden, which is an instant stress buster. But it's particularly beneficial for people with diabetes because grilling is also a healthy cooking technique. Grilled foods typically don't require high-fat sauces or accompaniments. And much of the fat drips away and never gets onto your plate. Here are a few ways to make your outdoor cooking even more healthy.

Skip the burgers and fill the grill with seafood and lean cuts of meat. You don't have to gorge on fatty burgers and sausages just because you're cooking outside. Healthier choices include skinless chicken breasts, beef tenderloin or sirloin, and fish.

Skin your chicken. Or you can leave the skin on while it's cooking to seal in moisture, and remove it off afterwards. It will save you from consuming a lot of saturated fat, which hampers insulin sensitivity and increases both calories and the risk of heart disease.

Bathe meats in a vinegar-based marinade. An American study found that taking 4 tablespoons of cider vinegar before eating a high glycaemic-index meal (one that includes foods that tend to raise blood glucose quickly) lowered the effect of the meal on participants' blood glucose by about 55 per cent. Low-fat Italian vinaigrette salad dressing with extra vinegar added will even do the trick. You can also experiment with your own marinades using vinegar, olive oil, wine, lemon juice, lime juice, garlic and herbs.

Get the most from your barbecue. Barbecuing may seem simple, but there is more to it than throwing on a few burgers or sausages and hoping they don't burn. Invest in a book of healthy barbecuing recipes. Variety is the spice of life and the more you know, the more fun you'll have. For a special event such as a milestone birthday or anniversary, consider hiring a chef. He or she can whip up a meal for your party and you will learn a lot, too. Ask the chef to focus on healthy foods that you don't know how to grill, say, salmon fillets, scallops or pork loin. The more excited you are about cooking healthy dishes at home, the fewer calories (and less money) you'll waste in restaurants.

make the change

The habit: Grilling fish instead of battering and deep-frying it.

The result: Less saturated fat and fewer calories consumed.

The evidence: A 100g serving of white fish fried in batter contains 231kcal and 12g of fat, 3g of it saturated. Grilled, without batter, the same serving of fish has only 112kcal and only 1g of fat (and no saturated fat). Making this easy switch cuts your calorie intake by more than half and eliminates the saturated fat, which hampers insulin sensitivity and increases the risk of heart disease.

whip it together!

Balsamic mustard-grilled prawn kebabs

You can't go wrong with healthy kebabs, which deliver maximum flavour for minimum effort. Vary this recipe by substituting scallops, cubed chicken, or lean pork for the prawns.

4 tablespoons **balsamic vinegar**

2 tablespoons **Dijon mustard**

1 tablespoon **olive oil**

2 tablespoons **honey**

2 chopped **garlic** cloves

2 chopped **spring onions**

450g peeled and de-veined large **prawns**

8 **cherry tomatoes**

8 **spring onions**, white parts only, cut into 2cm pieces

Mix the first 7 ingredients in a medium bowl. Cover and marinate for 1 hour. Drain the prawns from the marinade. On skewers, alternate 3 prawns, 2 cherry tomatoes and 2 spring onion pieces for each kebab. Grill over a high heat for 2-3 minutes a side or until the prawns are cooked through.

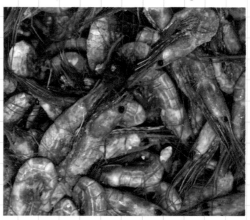

Skewer some vegetables. Many of your favourite fruits and vegetables taste better when grilled. Sliced aubergine, onions, peppers, mushrooms, tomatoes, pineapple, peaches and apricots all fare well on a grill. Coat vegetables with a little olive oil before grilling. For small or thin slices that might fall through the bars of your grill grate, use skewers or grilling baskets, which you can buy in DIY shops.

Grill delicate foods in packets. Barbecuing doesn't just mean chargrilled meat and corn on the cob. Packet cooking lets you cook all sorts of foods on the grill. Just put all the ingredients in the centre of a large sheet of aluminum foil, add a little olive oil or stock, then fold up the sides, leaving some room for steam to circulate inside. Set the packets on the grill. This strategy works particularly well for delicate or quick-cooking foods, such as fish and boneless chicken breast. Even lean meats stay tender. Put out a variety of vegetables (red or green peppers, onion, sugarsnap peas, sweetcorn, etc) and seasonings, and let each member of the family design his or her own packet.

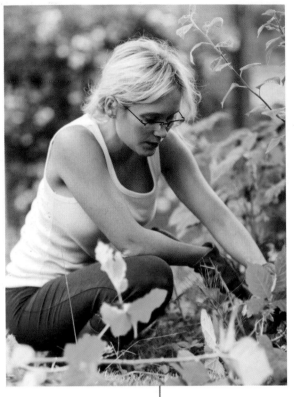

Put yourself to work

If you're going to exert yourself, you might as well get some fresh air and a beautiful garden in the process. What makes gardening so very satisfying is that, when you work at it, you – and your neighbours – will soon see the results. Abandon some of your 'convenience' tools in favour of some old-fashioned muscle power, and you'll burn even more calories while you work.

Make appointments with yourself to spruce up the garden. Make a list of every outdoor chore that needs to be done around your house. Break them down into 30-minute jobs. ('Mow front lawn', for instance.) Some of these jobs will be seasonal, and others will be monthly or weekly. Store this file where you will be able to refer to it regularly and add to it as you think of more jobs. On the family calendar, write in 12 to 15 jobs that are appropriate for the next month. You're more likely to keep appointments with yourself if you write them down.

Wash your car every week in good weather. In the summer there is no reason why you can't wash the family car once a week. In the hot weather it's a pleasant activity and, with the prices of professional washes as they are, it's a real money saver, too. Don't use a hose, though, as this is just a waste of water, and hardly any effort. You'll burn more calories by hauling buckets of water. Add to this all

---

golden rule

Use your knees to bend

Gardening and other outdoor work can be awfully tough on your back. When you need to lift something, always stand close to it and bend at the knees to pick it up. That way, your legs are getting a good workout, and you won't strain your back. Another way to protect your back is to carry a small stool with you to sit or lean on while weeding. You might also consider planting a raised garden bed.

the scrubbing and buffing involved and you can be pretty sure that you will burn around 200-300kcal per hour.

Skip the strimmer. Unless you have a garden that rivals the grounds of Buckingham Palace, a power-driven strimmer is probably more than you really need. Instead, tame the unruly grass blades that border your flower bed with a hand-held edging tool. Just be sure to keep the blades sharp, the mechanism lubricated, and wear work gloves to prevent blisters.

Rake your own leaves. Raking leaves can burn nearly 300kcal per hour. You get some exercise and you save energy (and money) by not using a noisy leaf blower.

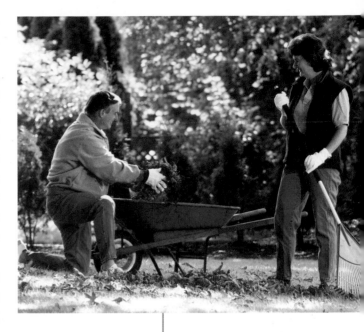

Sell your ride-on lawn mower. You don't have to push very hard to guide an ordinary electric or petrol-driven mower, but the walking will provide a nice low-impact aerobic workout.

Swing an axe to help heat your home this winter. If you have an open fire or a wood-burning stove, you can get some extra exercise by splitting logs and chopping sticks for kindling. Then you can light your fires the traditional way, using a bedding of sheets of old newspaper rolled diagonally, each one twisted into a ball and flatterned, with the dry sticks criss-crossed over them. Light this, then add some larger pieces of wood, then more when the fire is fully alight. Chopping wood to help fuel your fire will burn calories and you'll save money on firelighters, too.

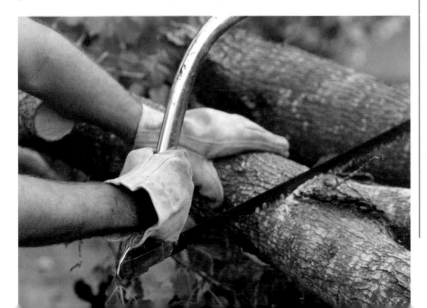

Cultivate a gardening habit

The outside of your house does double duty as a gym and a relaxation spa when it contains a garden. In fact, studies find that gardening is one of the best activities around when it comes to preventing or improving chronic health conditions. Aim for a minimum of 30 minutes of gardening (or other outdoor work) three to five days a week. You'll be controlling your diabetes and raising your property value at the same time.

Pencil in autumn bulb-planting on your calendar. Take the family calendar, go to one of the autumn months, and write 'bulbs' on three consecutive weekends. Plan for each bulb-planting session to last an hour. All that digging will give you a week's worth of strength training for your arms and shoulders, and your flowerbeds will look fantastic when spring arrives.

Do your own rotavating. When you start up a new garden, or if you're preparing an old one for new planting, break the soil up yourself with a shovel. If you're particularly ambitious and your garden is too big to till in one session, divide the job into smaller sessions or rent a mechanical rotavator, which will still exercise your arms. In either case, wear gloves to prevent blisters.

Pull weeds by hand. Give the soil in your flowerbeds a break from weed-killing chemicals. Instead, pull the invasive plants out of the dirt by hand. All you need are gloves, a hand-fork, a bucket or bag in which to discard the weeds, and perhaps kneepads. With your right hand, jab the fork tool into the earth at the plant's base to loosen the roots, and then pull the weed out with your left. Every 10 minutes, switch hands. The activity not only tidies your garden, it'll burn about 300kcal per hour for a 68kg person.

Plant a flowering showcase. Pick a flowerbed in your front garden that's prominent and visible from the street – this is where you will devote 75 per cent of your flower-planting efforts. Now give that bed the full treatment: well-fertilised soil; a newly installed, handsome border; carefully timed watering; and flowers selected for colour, height and season-long blooming. By hoeing, digging and carrying the watering can, you'll be getting an excellent workout in the garden and you won't even notice. To top that, the neighbours strolling by will almost certainly notice your plot, and you may even strike up friendships that you wouldn't have otherwise.

Bring your MP3 player outside for music while you work. Listening to music always makes arduous tasks seem easier. You can use the music to help you vary the stress on your muscles, too.

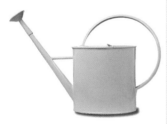

PLUS POINT
By hoeing, digging and carrying the watering can, you'll be getting an excellent workout in the garden.

Changing your tasks every four songs will help you to avoid putting too much stress on one set of muscles. For instance, you might start by pushing heavy wheelbarrow loads of mulch from your drive to the back garden, then switch to watering flowerbeds and so on.

Grow a healthier garden by keeping a compost heap. Compost heaps are good for the environment because they return biological materials such as grass trimmings and banana peel to the soil. But that's not all – cultivating them can give you a physical workout, too. A compost heap needs to be turned periodically to keep the rotting process humming along, which requires a little hoeing, raking, shovelling, or pitch-forking. You can burn off 250–300kcal in just 30 minutes of compost-turning.

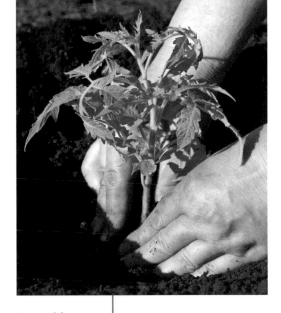

Turn off the sprinkler. The easiest way to water your garden is to set up a sprinkler, but that doesn't do your body any good. The next time you need to give your plants a lift, take a turn around the garden and aim the hose at each plant individually – not only will you be able to monitor each plant's progress more closely, but tugging and carrying the hose will do your muscles good. When this becomes easy for you, haul out the watering can instead of the hose. You'll know that your strength has improved when you're able to fill the can all the way and carry it with ease.

Plant your own 'locally grown' vegetables. Vegetables you grow yourself are as local, and as healthy, as you can get. You know that they're fresh as can be, and you know exactly whether pesticides or other treatments have been used on them. Successfully harvesting your own tomatoes, beans, lettuce, squash and other vegetables is also a point of pride. You'll be so pleased with yourself for having grown them that you're more likely to cook them frequently and experiment with new recipes, and you'll make sure that they'll never go to waste.

Plant a herb garden. There's no better way to add flavour to your meals than with fresh herbs, but they can be awfully expensive to buy. The solution? Grow your own. Culinary herbs tend to thrive in hot, dry conditions where nothing else seems to grow. Try sage, oregano, thyme, rosemary, tarragon and basil. For the most tasty herbs, feed plants only with compost, and water them as little as possible. This encourages compact growth and intensifies the oils that give the herbs their fragrance and flavour.

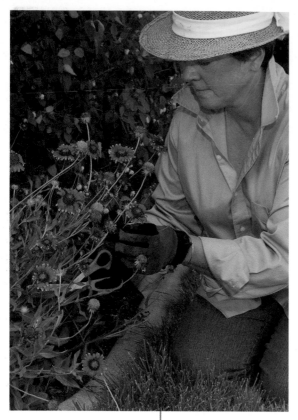

Protect yourself when you are working outdoors

Everyone needs to protect themselves from garden accidents, which are surprisingly common. But people with diabetes also need to make a special effort to protect their feet from blisters and injury, their skin from sunburn and their bodies from dehydration. Here's how to stay safe while getting exercise outdoors.

Wear breathable cotton trousers and long-sleeved shirts. Anyone who gardens with bare arms or legs knows how easy it is to pick up scrapes, scratches and insect bites. They're all injuries you might not have noticed otherwise, but they can get infected in no time. The answer is to cover up – but avoid very loose clothing that could get caught in machinery.

Always wear gardening gloves. Even moderate gardening will take a toll on your hands. Apart from scratches and nicks here and there, you're bound to get a few blisters. Buy multiple sets of gardening gloves and store them with your gardening tools and materials. If you're going to handle anything sharp – for instance, if you're changing the blade on your lawnmower – use heavy-duty gloves with thick leather to protect your palms.

Clear the ground before you begin. Before you start trimming hedges, pulling weeds and mowing the lawn, grab a bucket and stroll around the garden for 10 minutes. Toss into the bucket any debris that could cause injury while you work, including glass, stones, wire, sticks, nails and misplaced toys. All of these items can become missiles if a power tool hits them.

Rub on plenty of sunblock 30 minutes before going outside. Use sunscreen even on cloudy days. Choose one with an SPF of at least 25. A sunscreen that contains moisturiser is especially useful. When your skin is protected from damaging sun and kept moist, it's less likely to blister or crack – an invitation to infection.

Take action to prevent lawn-mowing accidents. If you have a push mower, mow across the face of any slopes instead of up and down the hill, and never pull the mower backwards. This will reduce

>> continued on page 106

Outdoor projects: exercise your options

Once a month, keep your body moving with one of these garden projects. To keep yourself focused, open your calendar and timetable these and other tasks months in advance – you'll be more likely to do the jobs if you write them down.

- **Install a stone border.** Pull up the rubber barrier that delineates the border of your flower garden and install in its place a handsome stone border. Your nearest garden centre will offer a variety of options in prefabricated stone.

- **Install stepping-stones.** Lay stepping-stones in your back garden, flush to the ground, following the most commonly travelled route.

- **Reorganise your shed.** Empty your shed and lay all of your tools and items on the lawn. Throw out everything that's broken or is no longer needed. Group similar objects together (garden tools, leaf rakes, car-washing gear, etc). If necessary, install extra hooks and shelving in the shed to accommodate these tools.

- **Rearrange the 'furniture'.** Devise a new look for your garden by establishing new positions for your lawn chairs, bench, picnic table, birdbath and planters. If you're great at plotting it all out in your head, fine. Otherwise sketch your plan on graph paper. It'll look like you have a new back garden.

- **Reseal the decking.** Depending on what your decking is made of and what kind of sealer you use, you may need to reseal it every one or two years to protect the wood from deterioration.

- **Reseal an asphalt driveway.** Experts disagree on how much protection driveway sealant provides. But two things are indisputable: a new coating will smarten up the look of your house from the street and it will provide a full afternoon's workout.

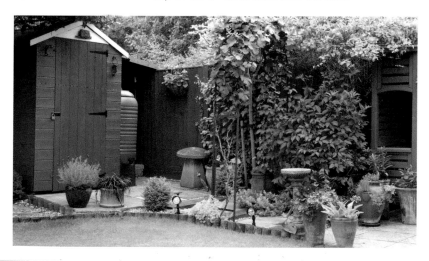

golden rule

Always wear shoes

Did you know that the spray from a power washer is powerful enough to cut through your toes? Without exception, you should always wear sturdy shoes – those with good support and rubber soles – any time you're in the garden to prevent falls and foot injuries. Bare feet, sandals and flip-flops are out of the question. Even on a well-kept lawn, there are just too many opportunities to step on sharp objects. Further protect your feet by wearing the right socks. If the nerves in your feet are damaged, the odds that a blister will develop and get infected are high because you may not be able to feel the blister developing. Look for socks that are seamless, have a padded sole, fit snugly without restricting your blood flow and don't wrinkle. Instead of cotton, choose man-made materials that wick moisture away from the skin.

the risk of slipping and being injured by the machine. If you have a ride-on mower, drive it up and down gradual slopes and avoid steep slopes altogether. Mow only in daylight, and make sure you can see a good metre or more in front of the mower. If your mower is self-propelled, never stand in front of it, and always disengage the drive clutch when you start it.

Drink extra water while working outside. To stay well hydrated, most people need a minimum of eight to ten 200ml glasses of water a day; when you're working outdoors in the heat, you should drink even more. Before you head for the garden, take a large jug and fill it with iced water. Park the jug in a prominent place so you'll remember to take a swig every 15 minutes or so. This will prevent dehydration, which can send blood sugar soaring. And drinking water keeps you from feeling hungry.

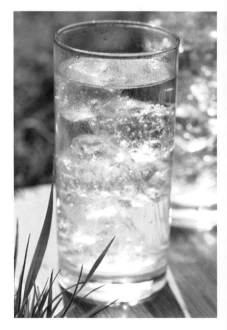

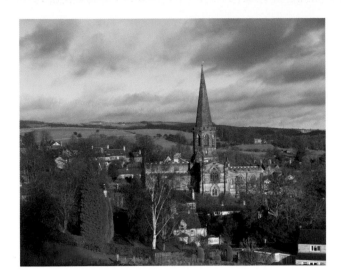

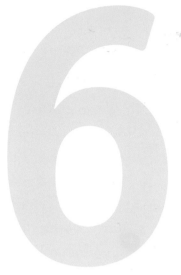

In your local community

Your community is much more than a

collection of houses — there are paths

to walk just outside your door,

friends to be made and

local resources to lean on.

Make the most of it all!

Step out

You don't have to climb Mount Everest to get fit; you can do it in your own neighbourhood. Recent research shows that getting 30 minutes a day of moderate physical activity can be as powerful as the best diabetes medications. Exercise boosts your energy and your mood and it increases your cells' sensitivity to insulin, which allows your cells to soak up more glucose and lowers blood glucose levels. Get moving with these simple strategies.

Walk the dog every day. Dog owners walk more than people without dogs. Not surprisingly, they also tend to be healthier, with less body fat, according to recent research. But not every dog owner takes advantage of these exercise opportunities. Those who don't walk their four-legged friends don't get the health perks. If you haven't got your own dog, perhaps you have an elderly neighbour who would appreciate you exercising his or her dog.

Volunteer at a local animal rescue centre to walk a dog several times a week. Some centres will be happy to have your help. Look on the internet or in your local newspaper or library to find details of your nearest centre and its opening hours.

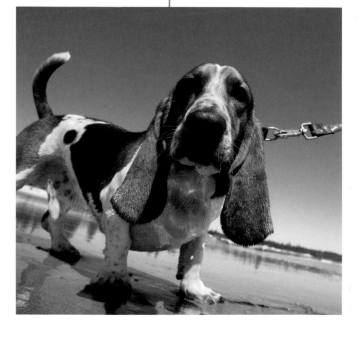

Sweep and weed your path once a week. Making a habit of keeping a tidy path in front of your house will make it more inviting to others, give you a chance to say hello to your neighbours while you're weeding – and burn off 100kcal in just 20 minutes of vigorous work.

Stroll to your local post office. If you have a post office within walking distance, make a habit of going there on foot instead of jumping in the car. And, if you are just posting letters, there is no reason why you can't walk to the nearest pillar box, whatever the weather. You will benefit from blood glucose-lowering activity and get to know your neighbours too.

Return wrongly delivered mail to its rightful home on foot. It happens to everyone: you receive a letter that should have gone to the house one or two streets away. Instead of marking it 'wrong address' and putting it back in the postbox, use it as an opportunity to stretch your legs, get some fresh air and perhaps meet a neighbour.

Take your newspaper on a daily walk. When you step outside for your morning paper, take the opportunity to go round the block. The fresh morning air will wake you up, you'll get a healthy start to your day with a few extra steps, and you'll knock 5 minutes of exercise off your 30 minutes-a-day goal before you even sit down to breakfast.

Use the pavement. Begin gradually, with a 15 to 20 minute walk. Stroll slowly for 3 to 5 minutes, then pick up your pace for 10 minutes and cool down for another 3 to 5 minutes. Each week, add at least 2 or 3 minutes to the faster portion of your walk. Within a few weeks, you'll be walking briskly for 30 minutes most days a week.

Try out a pair of walking poles. You'll burn far more calories on walks with these poles, which you use like a cross-country skier. It's called fitness trekking or Nordic walking, and using these poles can boost the calories you burn by 20 to 50 per cent more than ordinary strolling because the poles recruit the muscles in your upper body. Poles can also be helpful if you need extra stability or want to take some impact off of your legs. Follow the manufacturer's instructions for their use.

Say your ABCs out loud. When you're out walking, your pace shouldn't be so fast that you're gasping for air, or so easy that you can chat nonstop to your exercise partner without breaking into a sweat. If you're by yourself, recite the alphabet. If it's no problem, pick up your pace. If you start puffing by the letter F, slow down.

Score your exercise intensity. On a scale of 1 to 10, where 10 is running as fast as you can, and 1 is sitting on the sofa, aim for about a 6 or 7. At that level of intensity, you should be breathing harder than normal but still be able to carry on a simple conversation.

---

make the change

The habit: Walking 30 minutes a day.

The result: You'll live longer.

The evidence: Walking for half an hour a day can slash your risk of premature death by more than a third. Go a little farther, and you'll cut your risk by up to 50 per cent, according to a study that compared activity levels and death rates of almost 2,900 adults with diabetes over the course of 11 years. Researchers found that walkers lived longer than those who were sedentary.

Clip on a pedometer in the morning. The little gadget will keep track of how many steps you take that day – and subtly encourage you to take even more. Try to take 500 additional steps each week, aiming ultimately for as many as 10,000 steps a day. In case you're curious, 1,000 steps equal half a mile.

Keep a step log. It can take about six months for a change in behaviour to become habit. To help you maintain your walking habit, make a note of your steps after you take off your pedometer every night. Recording your progress helps you to stay focused.

Bad weather? Take an indoor walk. Go to a local shopping centre – one of the large, undercover types – and do a few circuits. The best time to do this is early morning or just before closing, so there won't be too many shoppers milling about. Do a few circuits, alternating one quick lap with a more leisurely lap. It's a great way to window shop!

Sign up with a local walking club. Most towns and villages have a group that organises walks in the local countryside. You can find details in the local paper, library or through an internet search. Do not assume that you have to be super-fit to attend; the groups are usually of mixed ability and welcome newcomers. You will be keeping active while meeting new people.

Join the Ramblers' Association. As Britain's largest walking charity, the Ramblers' Association has groups all over the country. Its website (www.ramblers.org.uk) has lots of general information about

golden rule

Stay safe on walks

In case of an emergency it's a good idea to pack a few items when you head outdoors. A backpack with zippered pouches and a water holder is perfect (you can find these at sports or outdoor shops). Always bring water and drink it at regular intervals whether you feel thirsty or not; dehydration can make blood glucose rise. Keep some glucose tablets in one of the zippered pouches. It's also wise to bring a mobile phone. Last but certainly not least, people with diabetes should wear some sort of identification – a medical ID bracelet or necklace or a tag on a watch – stating that they have diabetes and indicating whether they are on insulin or another type of medication that can cause hypoglycaemia.

walking and links to thousands of led walks going on every week. You can also download a free 'Get Walking Keep Walking' booklet containing a 12-week walking plan.

Use your car to measure errands you could do on foot. Put a sticky note on your dashboard that says 'Measure a route' to remind you to check the mileage to places you typically visit in a day. Is the library a mile away? What about the cash-point? People don't realise how many errands could be done on foot with a little planning, says Mark Fenton, an environmentalist and professional walking writer.

Grab your binoculars and go bird watching. You can pick up a beginner's birdwatching guide at a local bookshop. Look for one that includes birds in your region. It's a n intresting way to enjoy nature and connect with wildlife in the middle of your own community. Observing the beauty of birds and discussing them with friends, neighbours, or your children will add a new dimension to your leisure time. And interacting with nature tends to slow the heart rate, reduce blood pressure and help people to relax.

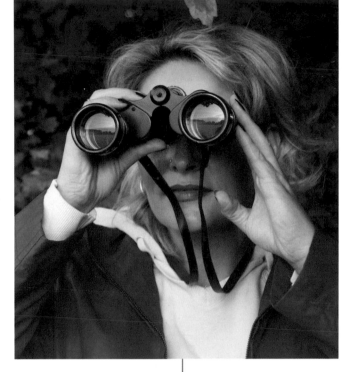

Put a 'Could I walk or ride my bike?' sticky note on the inside of your front door. Having a note in full view as you leave your home will remind you to ask yourself if you really need your car to take the books back to the library, pick up a prescription or visit a friend. Fix a second note to your dashboard that says 'Could I walk halfway?' so you'll be encouraged to park a few streets away from whichever errand you're on.

Organise your own treasure hunt. Whether you have kids, grandchildren, nieces or nephews, this activity never fails. Make a list that includes items such as five red cars, three houses with yellow daisies, two cats, four stop signs and so on. After you've compiled several 'treasures' for the kids to find, head out with them around the neighbourhood until you've found all the items on the list. You can make several lists and have friendly competitions. The first one to complete the list wins.

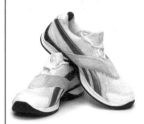

PLUS POINT
Ask yourself if you really need to hop in the car or if you could go by foot or by bike.

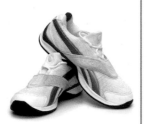

PLUS POINT
Walking shoes will encourage you to move more and will decrease your risk of injury.

Make after-dinner walks a regular habit. Instead of collapsing in front of the TV, create a household tradition of post-meal strolls with the family or your partner. If you have young children, you can play games to keep the little ones entertained. Remember the Alphabet Game during long family car trips? You can play it while walking. Look for signs, bumper stickers and personalised licence plates on cars, and watch for words that begin with each letter of the alphabet. Once you've found one letter, move on to the next.

Make a list of five active things you can do in your community. Hang the list on your fridge, and whenever you've run out of ideas for a weekend activity, take a look at it. For example, you could cycle to a local park to meet friends for a picnic, briskly walk to the library, or plan to meet someone at a halfway location to which you can both walk.

Have a monthly clean-up day. Grab a shopping bag and head outside for 20 minutes, picking up any discarded rubbish. You could even rope in a few neighbours to join you. After all, it's their neighbourhood too. Every time you have to bend to pick up a piece of litter, turn the move into a squat: extend your buttocks behind you and pretend you're about to sit in an invisible chair until your upper legs are almost parallel to the ground. You'll build leg muscles and sculpt your rear view. Building muscle helps the body to become more insulin sensitive, and it boosts your metabolism.

Lace up walking shoes for active living every day. You may think that any type of shoe will do, but footwear designed for walking will encourage you to move more and will decrease your risk of injury. A good shoe should be flexible in the ball of the foot, but not in the arch. (A shoe that bends in the arch can put strain on tendons in the feet.) The heel should be cushioned (because that's where your foot strikes) and also rounded to encourage an easy and speedy heel-toe motion. If you visit an outdoor or walking specialist shop, the staff will be able to help you to choose the shoes that best suit your feet and your walking style.

Burn calories at your children's football or rugby games. Instead of taking your folding chair and a crossword puzzle, wear comfortable shoes and take a stroll around the field during games when your child isn't playing. You can still cheer while in motion. Or take your walk before the game starts, when the children are warming up. Remember, physical activity enhances the action of insulin (the hormone that lowers your blood glucose), which often results in better blood glucose control.

Get to know your neighbours

The more sociable you are, the healthier you're likely to be. People who know others in their community tend to be less stressed and happier than people who live in isolation. Anxiety can raise stress hormones in your body that can in turn raise blood glucose and exacerbate insulin resistance. So use one of these excuses to get yourself out of the house or invite others over.

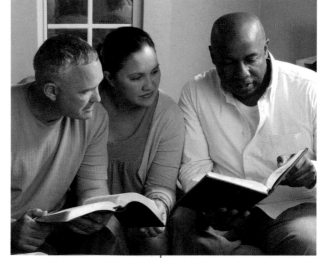

Have a weekly comedy night with the neighbours. Gather friends you know locally to watch a weekly TV show you all love and can laugh at together. Not only does laughing increase those feel-good hormones called endorphins, it also decreases blood pressure, pain, anxiety – and even blood glucose! A study from Japan showed that people who watched a comedy show after eating had lower glucose levels than those who didn't. If there's nothing funny on TV, take turns sharing your favourite funny movies with friends. If you're going to have food, save it for after the show so you don't unconsciously gobble up too many calories, and suggest that snacks be limited to chopped vegetables and fresh fruit.

Start a monthly book club. Network with your friends and neighbours to find interested members, or visit your local library, church, community centre or independent bookstore to post flyers

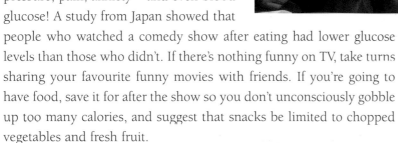

whip it together!

Picnic lemon rice salad

Bring something a little different this year to the gathering. A cool rice salad is just perfect for a summer picnic. Easy to transport and with a fresh lemon taste, it's a light dish that goes with any grilled seafood or poultry.

Combine 320g of cooked **brown rice** with 4 diced and deseeded **tomatoes**, 150g thawed frozen **green peas**, 1 peeled and diced **carrot**, 2 chopped **spring onions**, and a handful of finely chopped fresh **parsley**. Whisk together 3 tablespoons of nonfat **mayonnaise**, 1 tablespoon of **lemon juice**, ½ teaspoon of **lemon zest**, and **salt** and **pepper** to taste.

Add to the rice salad and toss well.

inviting people to email or phone you if they want to join. You can either have a round-robin arrangement where each meeting is held at a different person's house, or ask if one of the establishments mentioned earlier would be willing to host the gatherings.

Too busy to read books? No problem: buy or rent audio books. Listen to them on headphones during your walks, then get together with the group to discuss them.

Attend local residents' group meetings. You'll stay informed about local news, find volunteering opportunities, and meet others in your community. Check your local newspaper to find out when and where meetings are held. If you get involved, you might have a chance to promote local walking initiatives.

Log on to www.diabetes.org.uk to find local events. This is the website of Diabetes UK. Click on the 'In your area' tab on the home page for information about local diabetes activities.

Get on your bike. For journeys that are a bit further than you would like to walk, or to save yourself some time, think about cycling. If you fit a basket or panniers, you will even be able to carry a bit of

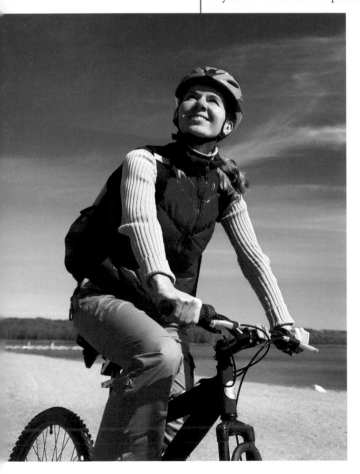

shopping. Make sure that your bike has been serviced and is roadworthy and buy yourself a cycle helmet and fluorescent strip to wear in the dark. At first you may need to push the bike up hills, but after a while you will be able to tackle them. Always listen to your body, and get off and push the bike if you need to; very soon you will feel delighted at progress you make as your fitness gradually improves.

Visit older people once a month. You can volunteer personally to visit a residential home, or volunteer through an organisation that organises visits such as Help the Aged, your local church or meals-on-wheels. As a volunteer, you will need to have a criminal record check, but once accepted you can become a visitor. Not sure what to talk about? People love to talk about themselves. Ask historical questions. Not sure what to do? Bring flowers, a book to share, a chessboard, some dominoes or a pack of cards.

Socialise the healthy way

Sometimes social events go hand in hand with calories and fat-laden foods. This is fine once in a while, but if you have a busy social life, you'll need strategies for protecting your blood glucose levels without sacrificing your social circle.

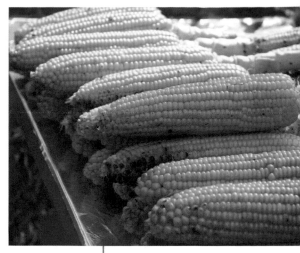

Examine the offerings before you fill your plate. It's all too easy to stuff yourself full of crisps, sausage rolls, pies and sandwiches if you just start piling things on your plate. But if you take a minute to look first at what's on offer, you'll make better choices. Avoid the fried chicken and choose healthier items.

Bring a healthy dish to barbecues and picnics. That will ensure there's at least one thing you can choose without straying from your eating plan. Try bringing a fruit salad, a tomato and cucumber salad, a juicy watermelon, or a platter of fresh vegetable sticks and low-fat salad dressing or hummus. For the grill, offer chicken kebabs with onions, mushrooms and cherry tomatoes interspersed.

Keep your hands busy at summer picnics and events. Stay away from temptations such as crisps and sweets by offering to be the official event photographer or starting a game of rounders.

Have only one glass of wine or one beer. Keep your alcohol consumption to one drink, since most studies don't show increased risks for a single glass. Avoid creamy cocktails as they tend to be loaded with sugar and calories. Don't drink alcohol on an empty stomach as it makes you more prone to hypoglycaemia.

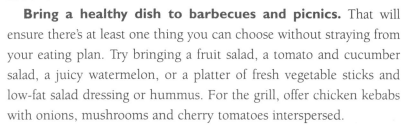

whip it together!

Mexican sweetcorn, chicken and bean pot luck

You might just have to plan on preparing a double batch of this simple, fibre-rich, one-pot dish as it will disappear very fast at a party. It can be prepared a day in advance.

In a large bowl, mix together 1 chopped **red pepper**, 2 sliced **spring onions**, 1 can (420g) drained and rinsed **black beans**, 1 package (300g) thawed **frozen sweetcorn kernels**, and 170g diced cooked **white chicken meat**. Whisk together 2½ tablespoons **olive oil**, 1½ tablespoons fresh **lime juice**, 1 tablespoon **red wine vinegar**, 2 crushed **garlic** cloves, ½ teaspoon **chili powder**, and **salt** and **pepper** to taste.

Add the dressing and toss well.

Fresh from your allotment

The very freshest fruits and vegetables come straight from the ground, and an enjoyable, inexpensive way to get more of them is to rent an allotment. For a relatively small yearly fee of around £25, you'll get a decent patch of land (9m x 6m), and the chance for as much exercise as you wish. Renting an allotment is also a good way to mix with people in your local community. You'll gain all the health benefits that come from socialising as well as from the gardening itself – digging, weeding, watering, hoeing and raking – which burns plenty of calories and builds muscle to keep you slim and lower your blood glucose. What's more, growing your own vegetables will encourage you to eat more of them, so ensuring you get the five portions a day that health experts recommend.

Where to begin

Take a look around your local area and you may be surprised to find that there is an allotment close to you, tucked in behind a school or on the edges of the railway tracks. It is a good idea to find one within walking distance of your and it will encourage you to get down to your plot regularly, preferably every day.

Once you have spotted a suitable site, you should apply to your local parish, district or borough council. If all the places are taken, you should be able to apply for more land to be made available elsewhere – if you can find at least five other like-minded neighbours. All councils in England and Wales (apart from Inner London) are legally obliged to provide allotments if approached by a group of at least six adult residents (on the electoral role).

Join an association

Council allotments have a steward in place whose job it is to allocate plots and deal with the day-to-day running of the allotments. But if you want your allotment experience to be more sociable, you should think about joining an allotment association (www.allotments-uk.com has links to associations across the country). Through an association you can swap gardening tips and save money by bulk-buying seeds and other gardening supplies.

No association close to you? No problem – start your own. First, contact all the allotment holders (perhaps via the steward) to see if there is enough interest. If there is, you will need to find a meeting place and set a time (try your local community centre, library, school or church hall; your new recruits should help you cover the cost if you have to pay a small fee).

Have a start-up meeting

At the first meeting, you can appoint a chairperson, secretary and treasurer for the next 12 months. The National Society of Allotment and Leisure Gardeners' website (www.nsalg.org.uk) has plenty of free, downloadable information about how to go about forming and running an association. Once formed, the agenda is entirely up to you and the group. Perhaps you can organise tool-sharing, seed buying and even watering rotas. The group will need to decide whether to seek funding and donations or to pay membership dues that would cover the costs of seeds, tools, fertiliser and other supplies. Associations can arrange talks, demonstrations and other events for their members such as a summer barbecue and a harvest swap meet, where you can trade a few of your marrows for some courgettes from a fellow plot-holder.

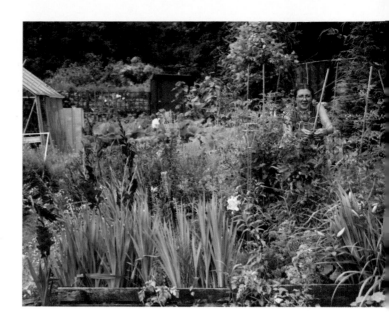

Homework before spadework

Once you have your plot, you will want to get to work, but take some time to plan your patch. If you're an experienced gardener, the chances are that you already know what you want to plant and when to plant it. But if you are new to gardening, you'll want to do some homework or ask the advice of an experienced friend.

Beginners' gardening books can tell you what typically grows in each season, how often you'll need to water and fertilise, how to prepare the soil, how to sketch a garden plot with what is to be planted where and what tools you'll need. There is also a good deal of information on the web at sites such as www.allotments-uk.com, which has articles on all aspects of gardening and a forum where you can post queries.

Prepare your plot and go for it

It's a good idea to break up the soil in autumn, and let the frost crumble it further. Mechanical rotavation will do this job and save a lot of aching muscles, but to get full benefit of exercise, you should turn the soil yourself with a spade. The golden rule for allotment gardeners

is little and often. Never do more than an hour of digging – you'll regret it the next day and may well be put off entirely.

Check what sort of ground-covering material is allowed in your allotment (some councils insist on biodegradable material available from garden centres, others don't mind old carpet). Then cover the ground, pulling back sections as you work.

As well as annual crops, consider planting fruit trees – you are usually permitted a certain percentage of permanent plantings adn are also allowed to construct a shed on your plot - very useful as it means you won't have to carry tools to and from your plot.

Enjoy your harvest

Perhaps the best part about working an allotment is the harvest, when all the hard work pays off. There is nothing quite like the taste of peas straight from the pod, or home-made blackberry jam. Once you have tasted how delicious home-grown fruit and vegetables can be, you'll never want to eat shop-bought produce again.

golden rule

Never let two days go by without exercising

Experts know that going without physical activity makes the body use insulin less efficiently, which in turn makes blood glucose harder to control. Researchers at an American university studying laboratory animals have now shown that when rats weren't allowed to run on their exercise wheels for two days, the amount of sugar taken into their muscle cells in response to insulin was cut by about a third. Whether or not the exact results apply to humans, the advice is the same: unless you're unwell, take some vigorous exercise at least every other day.

Make use of community resources

There are many community-based opportunities for improving your overall health, your fitness and your diet. Local papers will show you what's in your area. Here are a few tips to get you started.

Visit a public pool. There's no gentler place to start exercising than in gravity-defying water. Swimming is easy on your joints, burns plenty of calories and makes you feel like a child again, while giving you fitness and muscle tone. Because you weigh only 10 to 15 per cent of your land weight in the water, swimming or water exercise classes are good for people who have nerve damage that affects their feet and who need to avoid too much weight-bearing activity.

Enrol for resistance-training classes at a local gym. Resistance (weight) training is just as important as aerobic exercise for diabetes control. In fact, it's better than aerobic exercises at increasing insulin sensitivity, lowering your risk of brittle bones and preventing loss of muscle that slows metabolism. Group classes can be more fun, and safer, than using individual machines. Look out for bargain gym fees. Some gyms and leisure centres offer discounted rates for 'off peak' times, and if you are retired or unemployed.

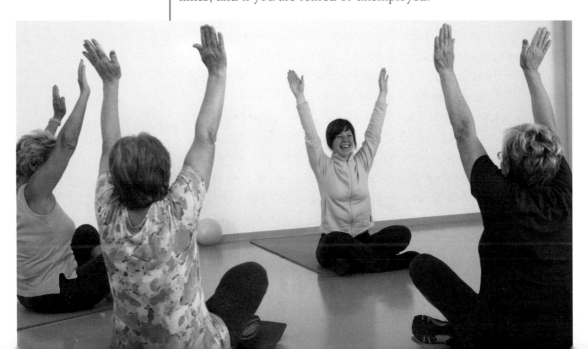

Invest in a personal trainer. Another way to tap into resistance training is to find a qualified personal trainer who has a local studio, works in your health club, or will come to your home. If you have weekly sessions for a month or two, you will be able to develop a personal programme that meets your individual strength requirements and fitness targets. You can search for a personal trainer in your area by asking at your local gym or by searching online.

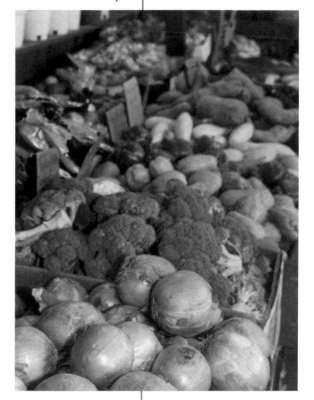

Take a healthy cooking class. Look for courses through local community colleges or continuing education courses. Go for general healthy cooking or sign up for a more adventurous vegetarian, Mediterranean, or Asian cooking class. It's a fun, productive way to get out of the house.

Make a weekly trip to the farmers' market. You'll find the freshest fruits and vegetables there, and also some interesting varieties that you won't find in the supermarket. In addition, the produce tends to be local and is often organic – which is good for the environment and your health. You may even meet other locals who are invested in community and good health. You can generally find information about local farmers' markets in your local newspaper, library or online.

Join a yoga class. Yoga is an excellent way to relieve stress. According to one recent study from California State University in San Bernardino, adults reported significant decreases in anxiety and increases in motivation and concentration after just eight weeks of practising a relaxing form of yoga, compared to a control group. Choose a gentle form of yoga such as Hatha that includes relaxing breathing. Most gyms and leisure centres now offer yoga classes alongside the more fast-paced aerobics and other fitness classes.

Pay a visit to a place of worship. Following their faith helps many people keep stress factors in perspective by reminding them of what really matters in life. Attending a local church or temple can provide a sanctuary from life's ups and downs that you can enjoy with others who share your beliefs. The same community can help you out and offer support during challenging times.

Volunteer to get out of the house

One of the best ways to improve your health is to help others. Whether it's at your place of worship, library or humane society, volunteering makes you feel good and gets you out of the house more often, increasing your activity level and improving your self-esteem. Helping others can lower your risk of depression, high blood pressure and heart disease.

Help out an ailing or elderly neighbour. Combine the obvious health benefits of exercise and fresh air with subtler 'feel-good' benefits that come from doing good deeds. Offer to mow the lawn, water the plants or walk the dog. Alternatively, bring round some library books, a few rented DVDs, or a home-cooked meal for your housebound neighbour.

If you have children, start a school 'crocodile'. As well as saving on petrol or bus fares, the 'crocodile' walk to school has the added benefits of exercise and socialising with friends and neighbours. It can be as informal as two neighbouring families taking turns to walk their children to school, or as structured as a route with several meeting points, a timetable and a regular rota. To get started, invite families who live nearby to do this with you, pick a route to your child's school and take a test walk. Then you will need to decide how often the group will walk together.

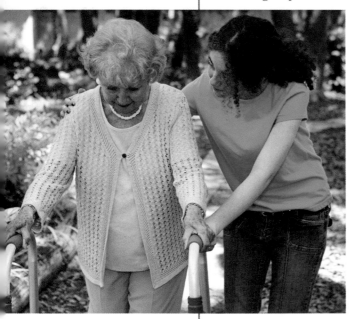

Volunteer to be a coach, referee or umpire for a local community sports team for children. Such sports clubs are always in need of this kind of practical help. Alternatively, you could volunteer to help with the warm-up sessions.

Help children learn how to read. Even if your children have grown up, your community is full of children who need volunteers to help them read at local schools. What better way to pass on your wisdom to the next generation? If you offer to volunteer at a school, be prepared to fill out some forms and have a health and criminal record check. Alternatively, you could help teach an illiterate adult how to read. Many libraries and adult education centres run volunteer programmes and offer free training on helping adults learn to read.

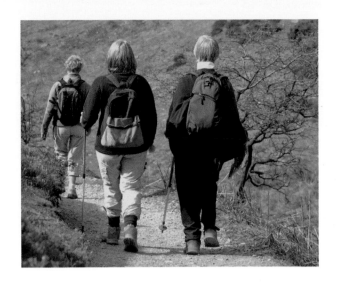

The great outdoors

As children, we ran ourselves ragged in

the garden, in the pool, in the park and

wherever else we could find to play.

We didn't think of it as 'exercise'

then, so why start now?

Get out of the house

and have some fun!

Keep it fun

You don't have to be one of those ten mile-a-day runners or a Tour de France cyclist to be an active person. Focus on sports and hobbies you love. Do them often, and you'll find yourself fitter – and maybe even happier – in no time. And it won't even seem like an effort.

Don't worry about aerobic versus strength training. Experts conclude that aerobic activity (walking and cycling, for instance) and strength training (lifting weights) are almost equally beneficial for controlling blood glucose, so pick whichever most appeals to you. Aerobic activity causes your muscles to burn energy and then draw glucose out of the blood to replace that energy, thus lowering your blood glucose. Strength training gives your body a larger mass of muscle, so there are more cells drawing glucose out of your bloodstream at any one time – another path to lower blood glucose.

Enrole in something fun. You might be turned off by the prospect of puffing your way around a running track or grappling with a series of weight machines at the gym, so appeal instead to the human desire for fun. Try a swimming-pool aerobics class that plays oldies music, sign up for tango lessons and dress for the part, join a hiking club to become one with nature, or volunteer to give walking tours at a nature reserve.

Invest in professional lessons, classes or retreats. You may do a double take when you find out the price of a three-day yoga retreat, but if you're going to splash out on something, your health should be at the top of the list. When you pay an expert to show you how to use weight machines properly, to ride a horse, or to belly dance, you'll master the skill faster and enjoy your pursuit much

golden rule

Choose an activity that makes you feel alive

People who play tennis every week, take a daily swim in the sea, or hit the golf course whenever they can don't do it for the exercise; they do it because they love it. (That doesn't mean it doesn't sometimes frustrate them to the point of throwing tennis rackets or golf clubs!) You may not love a new sport in the beginning, when your skills aren't quite up to scratch, so give it some time. But do choose a sport or activity you're naturally drawn to – that you simply think is fun or emotionally satisfying – and you'll be much more likely to stick to it and not view it as exercise.

more. And a few lessons is a small price to pay to ensure that you don't suffer any injuries.

Try a yoga or tai chi class. You don't have to work up a sweat to benefit from exercise. Both yoga and taichi increase your flexibility and balance. The slow, sure movements and gentle stretching not only benefit your muscles and joints but also your mental health – their ability to relieve

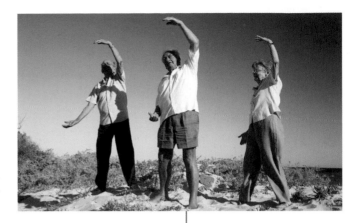

stress is proven. As being stressed can raise your blood pressure and drive your blood glucose down, or more often, up, those 45 minutes at the lesson can do you more good than you realise.

If you love people, keep it social. If you've got the gift of the gab or like meeting new people, seek out group activities such as bowls, tennis, squash or badminton. Staying socially connected is key to keeping your spirits up. You know what they say: laughter is the best medicine. If you are enjoying yourself with the people with whom you're exercising, the chances are you'll keep coming back for more.

Hang around fun, active people. If you have friends who love to hike or head for the driving range, their enthusiasm is likely to rub off on you. And most sports are more fun when you play them with friends. A study at the University of Iceland found that men whose fathers, brothers and close friends exercised with them (or who emphasised exercise in their own lives), were more likely to exercise and be fit than those whose friends and family did not participate.

Vary your activities. Your passion for any sport is bound to wane if you keep doing it day in and day out. Give yourself a break from your favourite game and do something different: go line dancing or hiking once in a while for a change of pace. If you always play golf, try visiting the local swimming pool once in a while.

Train for an event. Whether it's a five mile 'fun run' or a sponsored walk, put it on your calendar, then get out there and get ready. Give yourself plenty of time to work up gradually to the amount of walking or running you'll be doing.

Have a passion for helping? Volunteer to use your muscle. There are all sorts of opportunities for outdoor volunteers with many different organisations. You'll find a list at the National Council for Voluntary Organisations at www.ncvo-vol.org.uk. Your body will benefit and your spirit will, too, knowing the good you have done.

Exercise smarts

There's little or no excuse for people with diabetes to miss exercise because of their 'condition'. The fact is, people with the disease have scaled mountains, trekked across nations, won professional tennis matches and more. That said, it does pay to take some care when you're exercising. Start by following these tips.

If you have trouble standing, sit and exercise. Don't let limited use of your legs or unsteadiness on your feet stop you from getting fit. Buy an exercise video designed for people sitting in a wheelchair or chair. A good one will give you a heart-healthy aerobic workout and build your upper-body muscles as well. Such videos work well for people who are new to physical activity, even if they have full use of their legs. Many people are surprised to discover that they can work up a good sweat while sitting down. To get maximum enjoyment out of your sessions, find a video with an engaging host and upbeat music that will keep you moving.

Go easy on yourself if you're under the weather. If you've got the sniffles or have come down with the latest 'bug' that's going around, exercise only if you feel you have the energy and stamina to do so. If you don't feel up to it, give your body the rest it needs, and resume your regular exercise routine when you feel better.

Ease up if you're struggling. If you find yourself breathing heavily or if you're in pain or feel acute discomfort of any kind, you might be overdoing it. It's time to ease up. Give yourself the 'talk test': speak one complete sentence aloud. If you have trouble doing that, you should slow your pace. You should never feel pain, extreme fatigue, or severe shortness of breath.

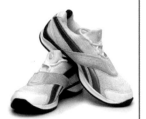

PLUS POINT
Exercise should be enjoyable. Stop, if you feel pain or suffer severe shortness of breath while exercising.

golden rule

Listen to your body

Because people with diabetes are at such a high risk of cardiovascular disease, it's important to tune in to what your body is telling you while you exercise. Stop exercising immediately if you experience chest, arm or jaw pain; nausea, dizziness or fainting (which are also signs of heat exhaustion or hypoglycaemia); unusual shortness of breath; or an irregular heart beat. All are signs of heart problems and should be checked out right away. For people with diabetes, the mantra 'No pain, no gain' definitely does not apply.

To speed your walking pace, take more strides, not longer ones. When you challenge yourself by quickening the pace of your walking or running, move faster by increasing the number of steps you take in a given time – not by increasing the length of your stride. It's more efficient and, if you lengthen your stride, the motion could injure your feet, knees or shins.

Buy shoes that feel comfortable as soon as you put them on. Don't tell yourself that your trainers will feel better when they're broken in. Ill-fitting shoes can rub your feet raw, which could lead to a dangerous infection. Whether buying shoes for tennis, walking, bowling or any other sport, choose the highest-quality shoe you can afford, and look for a model with ventilation that allows the shoe to 'breathe'. If you have reduced feeling in your feet due to nerve damage, you may need to consult a podiatrist about suitable shoes..

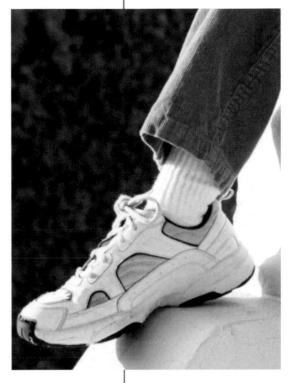

Wear soft, sweat-wicking athletic socks. Before you work out, pull on a clean pair of cushioned sports socks. Socks made from a cotton-and-synthetic blend are ideal because they wick moisture away from your feet. If your feet get moist, your skin will blister more easily.

Make sure your insulin pump's infusion set will stay put. If you wear the pump while you're physically active, apply antiperspirant or liquid bandage adhesive to the skin around your insulin pump's infusion set before taping it. This will help prevent sweat from loosening the infusion set's adhesive from your skin. Cover the infusion site with a small cotton ball, spray the antiperspirant on the surrounding skin, and allow it to dry before you exercise. The liquid bandage adhesive is available from online medical supply companies or from insulin pump companies.

Go to your GP with a 'frozen shoulder'. For unknown reasons, people with diabetes are particularly prone to a condition called 'frozen shoulder'. To test your shoulder mobility, try this: lie on your back on the floor with your arms at your sides. Raise your arm in an arc, as if you were doing the backstroke, and try to touch the floor behind your head. If you can come within several centimetres of the floor, your range of motion is normal. If not, contact your GP. Early treatment increases your odds of regaining full use of your shoulder.

>> continued on page 128

Exercising safely with diabetes

Having diabetes doesn't mean you have to avoid physical activity. It just means that you need to take more precautions than others do when you work out. Here's how to get on the road to regular physical activity and stay the healthy course.

1 Talk to your GP

Tell your doctor if you're planning to change your activity level. In general, becoming more active will do you good, not harm, as the benefits far outweigh the risks. However, if you have not been very active for a long time, or if you have had diabetes for some years (even if it has only recently been diagnosed), or if you already have some complications, your doctor will want to consider your physical condition.

Factors such as heart disease, kidney disease, nerve damage and eye damage must all be taken into account when deciding what kinds of exercise are suitable for you.

Discuss medication changes. Regular physical activity can lessen the amount of insulin or other diabetes medication that you require.

2 Learn when to test and when to rest

If you're on insulin, check your blood glucose before, during and after exercise. This is the best way to find out how the workout has affected your glucose levels.

Check your blood glucose before exercising if you have Type 2 diabetes and you're taking insulin or drugs that prompt the pancreas to produce more insulin. If your glucose is below 4mmol/l, make sure that you eat a carbohydrate-rich snack before exercising. During a period of prolonged activity check every 30 minutes to make sure your glucose level stays within your target range.

If you're prone to hypoglycaemia, check for several hours after exercise. This applies particularly to people who have Type 1 diabetes. Your muscles will continue to pull glucose out of your bloodstream, so taking a reading straight after a workout won't give you the full picture of your activity's effect on your glucose levels. You might think your blood glucose is normal while it's actually plummeting. Also, physical activity can speed up the rate that insulin gets into your bloodstream.

Time workouts to follow meals. If you find that you often have to compensate for hypoglycaemia by eating a snack during the physical activity, see if you do better exercising an hour or two after a meal.

As your activities change during the year, adjust food and medications. For instance, when the tennis season starts, you might be surprised to find your blood glucose running low if you don't account for the twice-a-week practices.

3 Be prepared

Keep essentials with you. If you're working up a sweat away from home, carry a high-carbohydrate snack, diabetes ID (bracelet, necklace or trainer tag) and a mobile phone for emergencies.

Brief someone you trust on emergency procedures. Make sure that someone in the vicinity knows that you have diabetes and what to do in an emergency. Whenever you're working out at home, make sure a family member is nearby; if you're at the gym, make sure a staff member is aware of your diabetes and would know what to do if you were unwell.

Wear shoes designed specifically for your sport. That means buying good running shoes for running, football boots for football, tennis shoes for tennis, and so on. It really does make a difference. Trainers with air or gel cushioning are a good bet because they will absorb shocks to your feet and knees.

Drink plenty of water before exercising. In the two hours before you start working out, drink at least two glasses of water.

4 Learn how to warm up and cool down

Start moving and stretching 5-10 minutes before intense physical activity. A warm-up can be a light-and-easy version of whatever activity you're about to start. So, if you plan to go running, warm up with a 5 to 10 minute walk and then do some gentle stretches to get your muscles ready for more vigorous activity. Weightlifting while your muscles are cold can cause injury; raise your body temperature first by jogging, riding a stationary bike, or walking on a treadmill.

Cool down gradually. As with the warm-up, do a brief, light version of your workout, keeping your arms and legs moving while your heart rate and breathing slow down.

5 Take care during exertion

Exhale during every lift. When lifting weights, exhale as you lift and inhale when lowering the weight. Holding your breath while lifting weights can raise your blood pressure. It can increase the pressure in your eyes and worsen eye diseases to which you may be susceptible, such as diabetic retinopathy.

Calories (kcal) burned per 30 minutes	
Cycling	272
Cross-country skiing	255
Gardening	170
Golfing (walking with clubs)	187
Hiking	204
Ice skating/roller skating	204
Kayaking/canoeing	170
Racquetball	238
Swimming	272
Tennis	238
Volleyball (casual)	102

Burn rates are for a person who weighs 10½ stone (67.5kg). Lighter people burn fewer calories; heavier people burn more.

Watch for symptoms of hypoglycaemia. It's easy to mistake symptoms of hypoglycaemia for the effects of exercise. The signs of low blood glucose include profuse sweating, rapid heartbeat, trembling, extreme hunger, difficulty thinking, blurred vision, loss of coordination and 'just not feeling right'. If you suspect you have hypoglycaemia, stop exercising immediately and consume a source of glucose, such as a glucose tablet or drink, boiled sweets or sugar cubes.

If you feel pain, stop exercising. If you start to feel uncomfortable or short of breath when you are exercising, slow down or stop. .

Drink water while you're working out. Experts recommend at least half to a whole glass of water every 15 minutes.

Don't exercise in extreme temperatures. If it's particularly hot or cold outside, find an indoor venue for your workout. In particular, be wary of hot, humid weather because it will be difficult for your body to cool down.

Comhairle Contae
Átha Cliath Theas
South Dublin County Council

On the court or course

Ask a golfer walking the fairways what he's doing. Chances are he won't say 'exercising'. Same goes for someone trying to perfect her tennis serve. Sports such as tennis, golf, biking and skiing are all suitable for most people with diabetes. Heed a few words to get the most out of them and make them safer and more enjoyable.

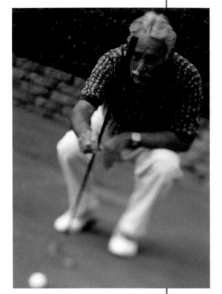

Take turns riding in the golf buggy. Walking for the duration of your golf match will give you the most aerobic exercise, of course. But some walking is better than none. If you need to ride a buggy at least part of the way, strike a deal with your partner to alternate who drives and who walks. For instance, you might ride in the cart while playing one hole, and your partner would ride during the next hole.

If you're playing all 18 holes, prepare yourself for blood glucose swings. Before you start a round of golf – or any other sport that will keep you moving for the better part of an afternoon – be ready with a glucose meter, carbohydrate snacks or glucose tablets, and any medicine you might need to keep your blood glucose in the safe range.

After squash, check for rising glucose. Don't assume that all types of exercise will lower your blood glucose. In some people with diabetes, high-adrenaline sports, or any very strenuous exercise, can actually raise it. That's because adrenaline causes the liver to release more glucose to supply the body with a burst of energy. The effect does wear off, of course, and you should be ready for a possible drop in blood glucose up to several hours after you've finished exercising. Regular testing – before, during and after exercise – will help you to determine how to manage your blood glucose levels with food, glucose or insulin.

Before a tennis match, inject insulin into your abdomen, not your tennis-playing arm. During heavy exercise, blood flow increases in the appendages that are working hard. If you inject insulin into a hard-working limb, the insulin will be absorbed into the body more quickly, and it may lower your blood glucose more quickly than you were expecting. The same goes for joggers – don't inject insulin into a leg before you set off on a long run.

Play on clay, not asphalt or concrete. Tennis can be tough on your hips, knees, ankles and back. The repeated impact against a hard-court surface can leave your joints sore and your feet battered. Asphalt and concrete courts are the worst offenders. Studies show that clay courts have the lowest injury rates – they're softer, allow a little sliding

>> continued on page 130

Choosing the safest sport for you

If you have diabetes, exercise is your friend, but you may need to choose between one sport and another if you have certain other health problems related to diabetes. Talk to your GP about your own personal health situation, but here are a few general guidelines.

If you have heart disease

✔ Good for you

Moderate, non-strenuous activity in moderate temperatures. Try walking, swimming or cycling on a stationary bike.

✘ Possibly unsafe

Straining and strenuous activity in very hot and humid weather or very cold weather. Avoid push-ups, sit-ups and walking up steep hills.

If you have peripheral arterial disease

✔ Good for you

Aquatic exercise, cycling and walking.

✘ Possibly unsafe

Weight-bearing and high-impact exercise such as basketball and tennis.

If you have high blood pressure

✔ Good for you

Moderate aerobic and strength training exercise. Walking, jogging and stair climbing.

✘ Possibly unsafe

Straining and strenuous exercise, such as power-lifting with weights.

If you have neuropathy

✔ Good for you

Moderate intensity, low-impact exercises in moderate temperatures. Swimming is a good choice if you have pain or burning in your feet.

✘ Possibly unsafe

Strenuous, weight-bearing exercises such as step aerobics, or hiking long distances and working out in extreme temperatures.

If you have retinopathy

✔ Good for you

Moderate, low-impact exercise without straining, during which you keep your head above your waist.

✘ Possibly unsafe

Anything that involves straining, jumping, holding your breath during exertion, or exercising with your head below waist level (basketball, heavy weight lifting and certain yoga poses).

If you have kidney disease

✔ Good for you

Light or moderate exercise (such as walking or swimming) and high-repetition strength training (using light weights and doing more than 15 repetitions at a time.)

✘ Possibly unsafe

High-intensity, vigorous sports and lifting heavy weights.

underfoot so there's less shock to the feet, and they slow the game down to a less hectic level. New synthetic court surfaces provide cushioning that protects your joints, too – you can feel the surface give underneath your feet when you walk on it. Natural grass courts (like those at Wimbledon) are softer but have a high rate of injury because the speed of play is faster on grass.

Make sure that your diabetes gear is secure when cycling long distances. Zippered pockets, a zipped-up backpack and panniers are good bets. You don't want to find yourself five miles from home on your bicycle and in need of a snack to keep your blood glucose up, only to find that your food has slipped out of your pocket.

Don't hang around on hot surfaces. If you have reduced feeling in your feet, make sure that you don't stand too long on sun-baked surfaces such as hard-surface tennis courts, concrete pool surrounds, asphalt and sand. Your feet could get burnt without you being aware of it, even through the sole of your sports shoe.

Can exercise reduce your need for medication?

Regular physical activity doesn't just help you to lose weight, burn fat and feel great – it can actually lower your cells' resistance to insulin, a core problem in Type 2 diabetes. The better your cells respond to insulin, the less medication you may need to take. If you're being diligent about following a new fitness plan and your blood glucose readings are showing a difference, it's worth talking to your doctor about whether you can reduce the number or quantity of medications you take.

Before your doctor agrees to make changes to your medications, he or she will probably want to study your blood glucose log and see how different combinations of food, medication and physical activity affect your blood glucose. The more details you can give your doctor about how you feel at any given time of the day, and what you did or ate before you took your reading, the better. A high blood glucose reading after exercise and a high reading after eating a jam doughnut mean very different things.

If you use insulin, ask your doctor whether and when you can substitute exercise for an injection, or at least reduce the amount of insulin that you take before a workout. Ask him or her how to coordinate your physical activity with your food intake, based on your blood glucose and insulin levels. Otherwise, you may run the risk of dangerously low blood glucose (hypoglycaemia) or dangerously high blood glucose (hyperglycaemia). Routinely checking your blood glucose before, during and after physical activity will help you gauge when you'll need a snack break or how long to wait to exercise after taking insulin.

Carry insulin and other essentials under your ski jacket. To prevent your test strips and the insulin in your pump from freezing while you are skiing, stash them close to your skin under your ski salopettes or jacket. One simple way to do this: wear shorts that have a secure pocket under your salopettes, and slide your insulin and test strips into the pocket to keep them out of the deep freeze.

Buy custom-fitted ski boots. If you love skiing and you have reduced feeling in your feet, buy your own ski boots and take care that you get them fitted properly. When you rent ski boots, your odds of getting an excellent fit are awfully low. And if you're wearing ill-fitting boots and you have reduced sensation in your feet, you might not realise that your feet are being rubbed raw. If you have impaired circulation in your feet, ask your doctor whether skiing could cut off circulation to your feet or put you at risk of frostbite.

Wear sunglasses with UVA/UVB protection. Good sunglasses will protect your eyes from glare as well as the damaging rays in sunlight, which can contribute to cataracts. Since people with diabetes are already 60 per cent more likely to develop cataracts than people who do not have diabetes, it's worth investing in a decent pair of 'shades' – prescription ones, if your vision needs correcting.

Carry a doctor's note that clears you for extreme sports. If you love some of the wilder sports such as white-water rafting, bungee jumping or skydiving, take along a letter from your doctor stating that you are cleared for the activity. The operators of such sporting facilities often will ask whether you have diabetes and may refuse to admit you unless you can provide a doctor's approval. Without such a letter, you may end up kicking your heels for a few hours while your friends have the time of their lives.

Join a team. Whether it's tennis, hockey, football, basketball, bowls or badminton that excites you, go on the internet and find a local team or league to join. Team sports not only boost fitness, they boost your self-esteem, too. Knowing you can't let your team down, means they're harder to quit than activities you do alone. And it's a chance to meet new people and make new friends.

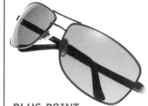

PLUS POINT
Always protect your eyes with sunglasses when exercising outdoors.

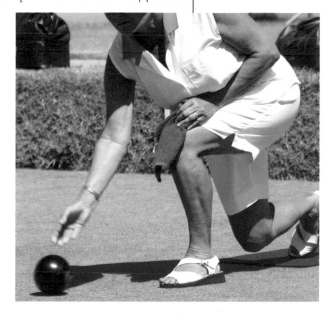

In the water

If you're overweight, or if you have joint or balance problems, foot pain from nerve damage, or other physical limitations – all of which are common among people who have diabetes – the swimming pool is one of the best places to get active. Because your weight is effectively reduced by 90 per cent in the water, swimming gives overweight people the buoyancy they need to keep their aerobic sessions going longer and move their bodies in ways they might not be able to do otherwise. Swimming is excellent aerobic exercise with an added benefit over walking: it exercises both the upper and lower body.

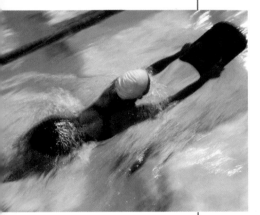

Splash in class. A water aerobics class may be the best way to get a full-body workout in the pool – and you don't even need to know how to swim. If there's upbeat music playing and you're with a nice group of people, you may even feel a little bit as if you're at a party. Want to get competitive? Find out whether your pool has a water volleyball team.

Get a leg up with a float. Your buoyancy in the water is already protecting your joints from impact, but if you need even more lift, a float or kickboard will help. They're also handy if you're not confident of your swimming ability and want extra help in staying afloat. People who just want to exercise their legs can grab a float by its sides and propel themselves through the water with leg power.

Work up to a 30 minute swim. Swim one pool length (25m in a standard pool) and then rest for 30 seconds. If that didn't challenge you, alternate swimming for 5 minutes and resting for 1 minute. Each time you visit the pool, add gradually to your swimming distance, resting as needed, until you reach 30 minutes of total swim time each session. To steadily improve your aerobic fitness, go swimming three times a week.

If your sight is impaired, ask about lane swimming sessions. Many pools set aside times exclusively for lane swimming, during which swim lanes are roped off and recreational swimmers splashing around are prohibited. Having your own lane reduces the chances that you'll collide with someone you couldn't see coming.

Protect wounds while in the water. Swimming when you have an open wound isn't a good idea because it increases your risk of infection. Rather than missing your aqua-workout when you have a cut or sore, ask your doctor whether a waterproof bandage or other type of skin barrier is appropriate for your situation. Be sure to clear the bandage with the pool's lifeguard or manager before you jump in.

Be extra-alert for low blood glucose symptoms. It may be harder when you're in a pool to tell if you're sweating or feeling weak – so be vigilant. Always take 'breathers' between lengths and get out of the pool as soon as you suspect a problem.

Get clearance to keep food near the pool. If your blood glucose drops while you're in the water, you may not have time to get to your locker to reach a snack. So keep a high-carbohydrate snack in a zip-close plastic bag by the pool while you swim. If food is banned from the poolside, talk to the manager and explain your needs; they may make an exception, or may let you keep glucose tablets handy.

Keep your insulin pump cool on the beach. If you're at the seaside or an outdoor pool on a warm day and you want to disconnect your insulin pump and swim, keep the pump cool so the insulin doesn't deteriorate. Place the insulin pump in a zip-close plastic bag, wrap a small towel around it and place it in a coolbag. Alternatively, check with your pump's manufacturer to see if it offers a special protective, waterproof pouch for your model.

If you swim with your pump, recognise its limits. Some insulin pumps are advertised as being 'waterproof' (sometimes with the use of inserts to plug the vent holes), but read the instructions carefully about the limits of this protection. The waterproofing may only apply to near-the-surface use and may not apply if you're diving more than a couple of metres underwater. If you find that the tape on your infusion set keeps coming loose in the water, buy a very lightweight wet suit T-shirt and wear that over the infusion set.

Protect your feet when swimming in a lake or in the sea – and even in pools. People with diabetes are prone to slower healing, and serious foot infections can even lead to amputation. Wearing water shoes or aqua socks when you're swimming in the sea will help prevent injuries from rocks, sea life, glass or other debris. Wearing protection in man-made swimming areas isn't a bad idea either; the concrete floors of some pools are abrasive.

Apply water-resistant sunscreen when you swim outside. The water may feel cool against your skin, but you could still get burned under the hot sun, even on overcast days. Sunburn is not healthy for anyone, but it's particularly vexing for people with diabetes because it can take longer to heal and, if it's bad, could possibly raise your blood glucose.

Shower immediately after swimming. Otherwise, the chlorine from the pool water will dry out your skin and might cause it to crack, which will make you more vulnerable to infection.

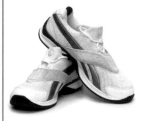

PLUS POINT
Wearing water shoes or aqua socks when you swim will help prevent injuries.

Pool exercise

There are plenty of effective ways to get an aerobic workout in the swimming pool without swimming a stroke – and your joints will be spared the pounding that they would suffer on land. Position yourself in a part of the pool where the water level is between your hips and your armpits. As you take steps during these exercises, place your whole foot flat against the bottom of the pool. Wear water shoes for better traction and to protect your feet.

1 Walking or running

The same movements that get your heart pumping on land will give you a workout in the water, too – with less danger of stumbling. **Bend** your arms at the elbow and **swing** them forwards and back as you go. Alternate walking (or running) forwards, then backwards.

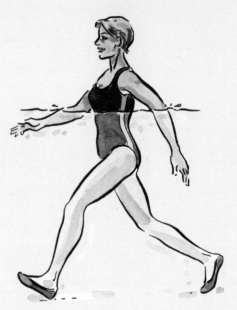

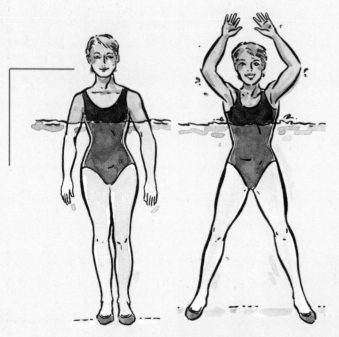

2 Star jumps

You might have learned this at school: **start** by standing in the pool with your legs together and your hands at your sides. **Jump** and **spread** your feet to shoulder width while you raise your hands up to touch over your head. Jump again and return to the starting position.

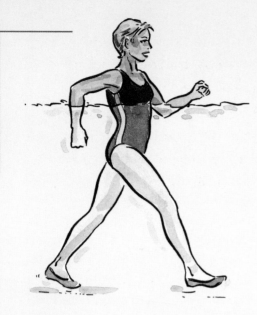

3 Cross-country skiing

This exercise is done standing in one place. Start by standing in the pool, with your right leg forward and your left leg behind you. **Hop** slightly and **reverse** leg positions – left leg forward and right leg back. **Swing** your arms forwards and back as you move your legs.

4 Front kick

Wrap a flexible foam tube around your back for extra support. Begin by standing in the pool. Raise your left leg in front of you, then return to the standing position. Repeat with the right.

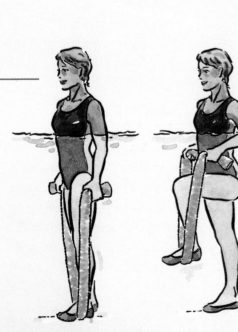

5 Knee lift

Stand up straight with the foam tube under your left foot. Bending the leg, lift your left knee to hip level, moving the flexible foam tube as you go. Return to starting position. Repeat with the right leg.

On your feet

Whether it's strolling on the beach that stirs your soul or walking every square foot of a flea market, moving your feet is doing your body good, so keep it up. If you're doing something you love, you won't even notice how much ground you're covering.

Visit flea markets and antiques shops. Grab your calendar and plan one day of leisurely browsing. Daydream about where you'd like to go, and make it happen: maybe it's ambling through a cluster of antiques shops that you've been meaning to visit, picking through the stalls at a flea market, or strolling up and down your favourite row of quaint shops.

Get lost in a large garden or gorgeous park. Maybe you can't resist inspecting every wild plant you see or snapping photos of the nature around you. Either way, terrific! Bring your hobby with you as your walk turns into a satisfying, stress-relieving outing. Don't forget to bring your binoculars and bird log if you're a birdwatcher.

Take a dog or a child along. If you're giving a dog a chance to run around outdoors or helping a child to enjoy nature, you're doing much more than mere walking. The time will pass more quickly and you'll come back with spirits lifted.

Mind your posture. Carrying yourself correctly can alleviate joint pain (and make you look thinner and taller). Stand erect with your shoulders back, your stomach muscles tightened and your chin up. Tilt forward slightly from the waist. Bend your arms at the elbow and pump them as you walk.

Calculate how fast you're walking and try to speed up. Drive along your favourite walking route until you have measured one mile on your car's mileometer. The next time you walk that mile, time yourself. (You might walk more than a mile, but this is where you can check your pace.) If you took 25 minutes, pick up the pace the next time and see if you can complete the mile a few minutes faster. As a point of reference, a 20 minute mile is considered a brisk walk.

make the change

The habit: Increasing walks to 90 minutes a day.

The result: Reduction of HbA1c blood glucose scores by 1.1 per cent – and possibly reducing the insulin or other medications you take.

The evidence: In a two-year study of people with Type 2 diabetes, those who walked for 90 minutes a day reduced their HbA1c levels (a measure of long-term blood glucose control) by an average of 1.1 per cent. The number who needed to take insulin fell by 25 per cent, and those who remained on insulin reduced their usage by an average of 11 units per day. Yes, 90 minutes is a lot of exercise, but shorter walks were also beneficial: study subjects who walked for 38 minutes a day still reduced their HbA1c levels by an average of 0.4 per cent.

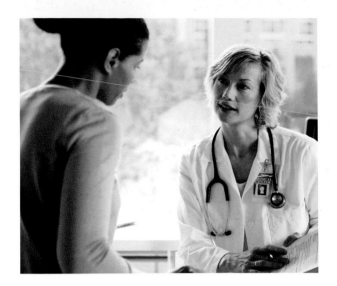

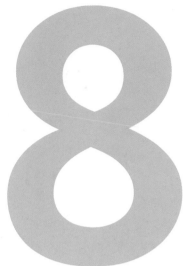

8

At clinic appointments

You're the one ultimately in charge of your diabetes, but health professionals are there to help – with medication, tests and their experience. The better your partnership with them, the better your diabetes management will be.

Working with your health professionals

Diabetes management is a team effort. You are the most important member of the team, but the various health professionals who provide services, education and medical care for diabetes also play a significant role. As clinic visits, tests and investigations become part of your life, it is useful to have some coping strategies.

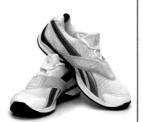

PLUS POINTS

Keep a note of what you eat, how much you exercise and any problems that arise; your notes will help when you discuss these issues with your team.

Get to know who's who. Whenever you go to appointments at clinics and hospitals you'll come into contact with a huge number of people. There's the receptionist who makes appointments and takes the basic information needed for your consultation, for example. Then you may see a health care assistant who might weigh you, take your blood pressure and test your urine. You may then see a doctor or nurse, who will discuss previous test results, and so on. It's worth asking each person what they do and how you can work together effectively so that you know exactly who to approach if you have any questions or concerns.

Keep the appointments. You'll be offered regular appointments at the diabetes clinic at least once a year (and usually two or three times). At least annually, you'll have an entire review, including physical examinations, blood tests and a consultation to plan your care over the next year. This will include a discussion of how often and how you will be in contact with the various health professionals.

For instance, you might have medical and blood tests and see your GP and practice nurse formally once a year, and in between attend education sessions with the diabetes specialist nurse and dietitian. You will also be offered a retinal screening appointment. Whatever is set out in your annual care plan should be written down so that it is clear to everyone.

It's important to attend the appointments and sessions you plan together; research shows that people who keep to their care plan fare better than those who don't. If you need transport to appointments, or help with costs, your clinic should be able to assist you with these.

Know your blood glucose targets

Your blood glucose level will vary from hour to hour and day to day, depending on your activity, food intake, medication and how you're feeling. It is only considered too high if it is consistently above the recommended range. An occasional day or two, or the odd test outside the recommended range is acceptable. All blood glucose targets should be personal ones, but Diabetes UK give the following guidelines:

▶ **Generally speaking**, blood glucose levels should be between 4 and 6mmol/l before meals and less than 10 mmol/l two hours after a meal.

▶ **High blood glucose:** too high is anything consistently over 10mmol/l.

▶ **When to seek help:** if you are experiencing fluctuating levels, or if changes you have made to your medication, activity or food have not made a difference to your blood glucose levels and they are consistently higher than the levels recommended for you, then get in touch with your GP or practice nurse.

Voice any concerns about your care plan. Speak up if for any reason you are worried about the recommendations and expectations of your health care professionals — for example, if your feet burn so much that you can't exercise, if you are terrified of needles and don't think you'll be able to inject yourself with insulin, or if there's nowhere to keep your insulin cool on holiday. These are all problems that your team can help you to solve or work around.

Bring your test results diary and food diary if you have them. Both can help you to have a more useful consultation with your health professional, whether it is your doctor, practice nurse or dietitian. A second pair of eyes on your information might help you to identify a trend that you have overlooked, or notice where you're consuming the extra calories that make it so difficult to achieve your weight-loss target.

Bring helpful extras. Other useful items to have to hand during appointments are your reading glasses, if you wear them, and a list of all your current tablets and other medications. Be sure to include over-the-counter preparations and any herbal or vitamin supplements you are taking.

Bring an extra set of ears. It can be difficult to take in everything that is said during a consultation. As well as making sure that you don't miss anything important that your health professional tells you, a friend or relative can remind you of all the questions you wish to ask.

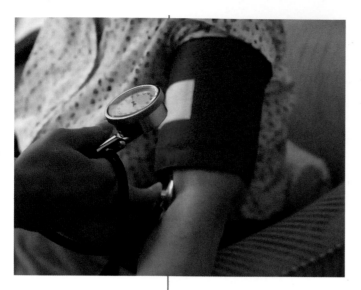

Sometimes clinic appointments may be more stressful than you expect and your companion will be able to provide emotional support. If you wear a hearing aid, make sure that you take it with you.

Wear comfortable clothing and shoes that can be easily removed. It may sound obvious, but if you are attending an appointment that requires medical tests such as a foot examination, blood pressure check or ECG (a painless measurement of your heart rhythm, but one which involves leads being attached to your chest and arms), then wearing light trousers and tops and slip-on shoes can save time not to mention dignity.

Take a few deep breaths before you have your blood pressure checked. This simple strategy can help you to relax so that any of your normal feelings of nervousness or apprehension about attending the appointment won't interfere with your test results, and your blood pressure reading will be as accurate as it can be.

Ask what your blood pressure is. You should be told the reading and have it written in your notes, but sometimes it may be overlooked, or you may just be told that it is 'normal' or 'a bit high'. Since your blood pressure is such an important indicator of your condition, you need to know precisely what it is. So speak up and ask for the exact reading. Ideally, blood pressure for people with diabetes should be 130/80 or lower. If your pressure is consistently higher, it indicates the need for you to have treatment that will lower it to within the recommended range. Excessively high blood pressure over time leads to an increased risk of heart disease and stroke, as well as nerve and kidney damage.

Learn how to get help out of hours. Is there an alternative number you should call? Who are the other doctors who will be on call when your doctor is away? Which out-of-hours clinic should you use? Ask these questions before a crisis strikes.

Does your doctor have a blind spot?

If your doctor has a computer in the consultation room and you find that he or she spends more time looking at your case notes on screen than at you, you need to take action. Ask politely if you can have a face-to-face discussion, and raise any issues that concern you.

Before your appointment

You probably go to the clinic only a handful of times each year, so make the most of those visits with a little advance preparation. It could pay off later by eliminating the hassle of having to repeat an appointment because of a missed blood test or because you forgot to ask an important question.

Make a list of questions. Appointments go by so fast that it's hard to remember everything you want to ask or discuss unless you write it down. Let the person who you are seeing know that you have been thinking about your diabetes and would like to ask questions. To make sure you keep track of everything you want to ask, number or bullet each item on your list, leave space to take notes and tick off each item after you've talked it over. That way, even if there isn't time for all your questions, you'll be able to refer back to your notes and know what still needs to be discussed.

Get blood tests done in plenty of time before your visit. Your clinic may ask you to have tests prior to your appointment. If you wait until the last minute, you may not get the results in time.

Get detailed instructions about any future tests. Find out if you'll need to make an appointment, or if they have walk-in times. Will you need to fast and, if so, for how long prior to the visit? If it's an exercise stress test, what should you wear? Do you need to have the tests and investigations completed a certain number of days before your appointment?

Review what you eat. If you're not careful, you can 'out-eat' the effectiveness of most diabetes drugs. Before your next visit, take an honest look at your diet and ask yourself if you're doing everything you can to eat more healthily. At what times of day do you generally eat? (Many diabetes medications are more effective when properly timed with meals.) How often do you eat out? (It's much harder to keep calories under control when you eat out.) What are your portion sizes? Do you limit sugary or high-fat foods? At your appointment, you will probably be asked about what you eat and when you eat it. Thinking about it in advance can make this conversation more useful.

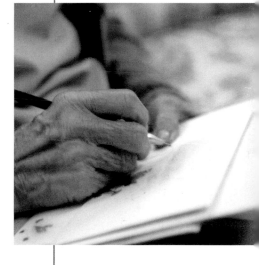

Maintain your normal diet before blood tests. That is, unless your doctor told you to fast. (If you're not sure, ask.) If you're eating or drinking habits were out of the ordinary on the day of a blood test or other investigation, be sure that you tell your doctor as this could affect the results.

Questions to ask

Going to clinic appointments can be stressful and sometimes the consultations are quite short, so it's not uncommon to feel a bit rushed. But do ask your questions. Getting the answers you need makes the difference between taking good care of your diabetes, and your health in general, and letting it slip from your control. Start with the tips offered here.

How often should I check my blood glucose? The answer will depend on several factors. See the explanatory panel on page 148. At each visit, you'll want to review and discuss how you are using your monitoring results at home and whether you should increase or decrease the frequency of your tests.

How and when do I take my medications? This is crucial, and the instructions for you might be different than for somebody else, so pay careful attention and take notes. Make sure you know if you should take your medication or insulin before or after meals, at night or in the morning, with or without food, and so on. Do you need to avoid alcohol? Are there potential interactions with other drugs that you should know about? This information will be included when you pick up your prescription, but the language can be hard to understand, so it doesn't hurt to ask while you're at the clinic.

Could I take longer-acting versions of my tablets? New formulations of tablets are constantly coming on to the market, and taking a longer-acting formulation might reduce the number of tablets you need to take each day, so it is worth asking for an update on what is currently available.

What side effects could I experience? Any prescription you receive should come with a leaflet that describes possible side effects and symptoms, but it's a good idea to discuss these issues when your medications are first prescribed. Are some side effects more likely than

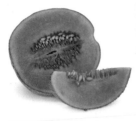

PLUS POINT

Cantaloupe is rich in vitamin A. It helps to protect you from some of diabetes' major complications.

See your doctor as an equal

The certificates and diplomas on a doctor's wall can be both impressive and intimidating – but does he or she know how to change a spark plug, prepare a gourmet meal, speak a second language or paint? Remind yourself of your own special talents which may be different but are no less valuable. One person is not better than the other. Keep this in mind and you may not be as intimidated or shy about asking questions.

others? Will the medication make you drowsy or unable to drive a car? What symptoms warrant a call to the doctor? Should you stop taking a drug if you experience certain unpleasant effects? If for any reason you do stop taking a medication, let your clinic know promptly. Don't wait for the next appointment.

What sort of eating plan should I follow? You will have the opportunity to discuss food and your eating plan in detail with a registered dietitian, but if you have questions about what to eat in the meantime, your GP or practice nurse will be able to help. Typically this will involve not skipping meals, eating at the same times of day every day, eating similar amounts of food at a given mealtime, and focusing on fresh fruits and vegetables, whole grains, low-fat dairy and lean protein foods.

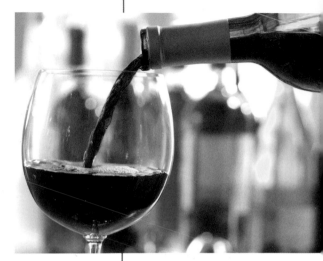

Can I drink alcohol? The general rule is a maximum of 2 units of alcohol a day for women and 3 a day for men. (One unit is half a pint of beer, a small glass of wine or one measure of spirit.) If your tests indicate problems with your kidneys or your liver, your doctor may suggest that you reduce your intake or avoid alcohol altogether.

Should I avoid certain foods? Based on your blood pressure, cholesterol and blood glucose averages, you may need to alter your diet. The prevailing school of thought is that you can still eat most of the foods you enjoyed before being diagnosed with diabetes, including sweets, though maybe not in the same amounts or prepared in the same way. For example, if you have been having a lot of sugary fizzy drinks to quench your thirst, you will need to switch to diet or low-calorie versions.

Can I go to salsa classes or play tennis? As long as you don't have serious health complications, most doctors will recommend moderate exercise such as walking, swimming or riding a bike for 30 minutes most days a week. Still, it is a good idea to get the go-ahead if you're starting a new physical activity or exercise regimen. You may need a health check, for example, if you have kidney disease, nerve damage, signs of heart disease or other problems,.

Can I reduce any of my medications? This is a perfectly valid question to ask if you've been eating healthily and exercising regularly, and you've seen significant improvements in your blood glucose levels as a result.

Diabetes medications

Healthy eating and regular physical activity will always be critical for keeping your diabetes under control – but it won't always be enough. There will probably come a time, if it hasn't come already, when you will also need tablets or insulin to help you to control your blood glucose. Here are a few ideas on what you can expect.

Who needs drugs?

If you have Type 2 diabetes, at first you will be advised to bring down your blood glucose with healthy eating and regular exercise, but relatively few people can avoid medication completely by these means alone.

If your blood glucose levels are extremely high without an obvious cause (such as drinking a lot of sugary drinks), you may be asked to take tablets straight away, even if this is temporary. You may also be prescribed drugs early on if you are not overweight (about 10 per cent of people with Type 2 diabetes are a healthy weight), or if you are already eating and exercising according to recommendations.

Even if you don't fall into one of these categories, it's becoming common for doctors to prescribe an oral drug such as metformin immediately. (According to estimates, most people have had diabetes for at least five years before they are diagnosed, so this makes sense.)

Even if you don't start off using medications, many people will eventually need drug therapy. The longer you have diabetes, the harder it is to manage it with diet and exercise alone because it is a progressive condition.

What about insulin?

Sometimes it makes sense to use insulin straight away. This is essential if you have Type 1 diabetes, extremely high blood glucose levels at the time of diagnosis, if you have severe liver or kidney damage, or have a greater need for insulin due to illness or stress. Still, most people with Type 2 diabetes start with one or two oral medications. If it becomes obvious that diet, exercise and pills aren't working, you and your health professionals may decide that it's time for insulin. If you need insulin injections, you will be able to learn the necessary skills involved from your diabetes specialist nurse or practice nurse.

What medications might I need?

There are a handful of different kinds of diabetes drugs available, and they can be used alone or in combination, depending on what sort of help your body needs to control your blood glucose. Some drugs work on the pancreas to help your body secrete more insulin; some lower the amount of stored glucose released from your liver; some lower your cells' resistance to insulin; some help your body to release a quick burst of insulin when you eat; and some slow down the rate at which carbohydrates reach your bloodstream after a meal. Certain drugs, called sulphonylureas, can cause weight gain, so your doctor may avoid prescribing one of these if you're overweight. Your doctor will also consider your kidney function. For example, drugs that are eliminated from the body through the kidneys, such as metformin, may not be a good choice for you if you have kidney damage.

Why might my dose or drug be changed?

Type 2 diabetes is progressive, so over time you may need additional, or higher, doses of your medication. An illness or stressful life event, might also mean that you need increased doses or the addition of insulin to your tablets. All doses and new medications are 'provisional', to see if they suit you and have the desired effect.

What about side effects?

In general, diabetes medications are safe and work well. But like any other drugs, they have potential side effects. Discuss each of your medicines with your health professional, and read the package insert carefully. Any drug can interact with other medicines – prescription or otherwise – and some diabetes tablets do not sit well with alcohol, so be sure to get good directions and heed them. Common side effects of some drugs are hypoglycaemia, stomach upset, skin reactions, bloating and weight gain.

Most are mild and temporary, but there is a formal reporting system for side effects, so if you experience any, do discuss them at an early stage with your GP or diabetes specialist. If media reports about drugs you are taking are causing you any concerns, make some notes and check with your pharmacist or other health professional to decide the best course of action.

Drug treatments for Type 2 diabetes
*Based on NICE guidelines issued May 2008.

Your doctor's approach may vary according to your personal situation. All these treatment steps include healthy eating and increased physical activity.

Situation/ *HbA1c level	Likely Treatment/Approach	Comments
At diagnosis and for first 3 months	Attention to healthy eating, losing weight if needed and increasing aerobic physical activity to at least 30 minutes a day.	Metformin may be prescribed at an earlier stage, to help weight loss.
Higher than 6.5%	Metformin tablets, dose stepped up gradually over several weeks. Addition of sulphonylurea if high HbA1c persists.	Sulphonylurea may be used if you're not overweight or can't tolerate metformin. Sulphonylureas can cause weight gain and hypoglycaemia: you should be given clear, practical guidelines to manage this.
Higher than 7.5%	Add a thiazolidinedione or insulin.	Exanatide may be used according to certain criteria, e.g. very overweight, weight causing psychological problems.
Consistently higher than 7.5%	Start and/or increase insulin, changing doses and formulations over time to achieve blood glucose targets.	Particular combinations of tablets and insulin, or insulin formulations, and doses will depend on the individual.

*Your Haemoglobin A1c (HbA1c) level, measured by a blood test, indicates the trend of your blood glucose levels over the past 8-12 weeks. (See page 151)

Share your symptoms

You may be reluctant to reveal certain details – hiding a swollen toe under a sock, or 'forgetting' to mention embarrassing new problems. It's essential to speak up because what seems like harmless indigestion, a 'floater' in your eye, or tingling in the feet may indicate something more serious, but at a stage when it can be successfully treated.

Be clear when explaining symptoms. Instead of just saying 'I've been feeling lousy', try to be as specific as possible. For example, 'I've been feeling a tingling in my feet for the last two weeks'. Describe your symptoms as precisely as possible, say what you've been doing to relieve them (if anything), and note whether anything seems to help. The more specific you are, the easier it will be for health professionals to work out with you a diagnosis and treatment.

Report any tingling, numbness, burning or pain. These sensations in your feet, legs, arms or hands can be a sign of nerve damage or neuropathy. The feelings often start in the feet and can be slight at first. Give a description of any sensitivity to touch, leg cramps, difficulty sensing the position of your feet, or feelings of being off-balance. Other markers of circulation and nerve problems in the feet are sores, blisters or cracks that won't heal.

Scale your pain. It might be helpful to tell your doctor how much pain or discomfort you are in by using a scale of 1 to 10, where 10 is excruciating pain and 1 is very mild discomfort.

Share even embarrassing symptoms. While you may feel uncomfortable talking about frequent urination or erection problems, health professionals often hear about these and know how to help.

Know the signs of high and low blood glucose

Common signs and symptoms of hypoglycaemia (low blood glucose) are confusion, hunger, weakness, shakiness, rapid heart beat, perspiration, dizziness, nervousness or irritability. Signs and symptoms of hyperglycaemia (high blood glucose) include fatigue, thirst, frequent urination, blurry vision, hunger and weight loss. You won't necessarily have all the symptoms at once, and they can vary from episode to episode. Some people report unusual symptoms such as their nose going numb or their ears ringing. If you experience any of these, discuss them with your doctor.

Learn to monitor your blood glucose

The whole point of taking medications, eating healthy foods and taking exercise is to keep your blood glucose within reasonable targets – and there's no way of knowing how well these steps are working without checking your blood glucose regularly. The more often you test, the better you can focus on the perfect combination of strategies.

Master the self-test. Your GP, practice nurse, pharmacist or diabetes specialist nurse (whoever supplies your blood glucose meter) will show you how to test your own blood glucose. You'll start by preparing the meter and test strip, and then you prick your finger with a small needle, called a lancet. Some meters have a built-in lancet that takes blood from your forearm or thigh, and there are also spring-loaded lancing devices that resemble a pen and make pricking yourself easier. If you use your fingertip, prick the area beside your fingernail to avoid having sore spots on your finger pads. Apply the drop of blood to a testing strip. Your meter will provide results in about 5 to 30 seconds, and you can record the numbers in a log book; all modern meters also record and store the results.

Know when you should check blood glucose. Everyone's timetable will be different. See 'How often should I check my blood glucose?' on the following page.

Discuss blood glucose testing with your health professionals. Talk to the staff at your clinic or at the pharmacy about the many different meters available. The strips they use are not interchangeable, although they are available on prescription. To make sure you get the right meter for you, ask to see a range. You may be able to try out different meters through your diabetes clinic. You can also talk about the advantages for you of doing regular self testing.

Know what to do with the results of your blood glucose test. This is vitally important, as there is no point at all in testing and recording your glucose levels if you are not able to take any action on the results. How to interpret different levels is an important part of your education when you are first learning about testing. For example, what you should do if your level is higher or lower than the recommended figure for you (usually in the region of 4-6mmol/l before meals and up to 8mmol/l after meals) for a set period. Discussing what action to take is an integral part of teaching you how to manage your diabetes successfully.

Address high morning blood glucose. During the early hours of the morning, the body secretes hormones that inhibit insulin so that more glucose is available to the body at the start of the day – not what

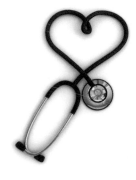

PLUS POINT
Discover your danger zone. Ask your doctor what blood glucose level is too high and might be an emergency.

you need if you have diabetes. If your blood glucose drops too low in the middle of the night, a related phenomenon can occur, causing your body to react – actually, to overreact – by releasing hormones that raise blood glucose. If you notice a pattern of high morning blood glucose, you may need to change the type or dosage of medication or insulin you take, or when you take it, or tweak your evening eating habits. Your blood glucose will be easier to manage throughout the day if you can start the day off with normal readings.

Know when you might need to check more often. You'll want to do extra checks when you're unwell or under significant stress. You may also need to do extra checks when you make a change to your treatment plan.

How often should I check my blood glucose?*

The point of checking your blood glucose is to see what effect the foods you are eating, the medications you are taking and the exercise you are doing have on your levels, so you can tell how well they're working. Testing regularly and at different times will give you useful information.

▶ **If you aren't taking oral medications or insulin,** your blood glucose level is likely to be measured using 3-6 monthly HbA1c tests (the target range is 6.5-7.5%). If your HbA1c is high, your levels are very variable or your treatment is changing, you may be asked to do some home blood glucose tests. If you wish to see the effects of the changes you are making to your food intake and activity levels, you can choose to do self testing. Discuss your needs with your health professional.

▶ **If you are taking oral medications,** you may be asked to test yourself once or twice a day at different times, especially when you have started a new type of tablet or are taking a new dose. Test more often if you are changing your physical activity levels or you are ill.

▶ **If you take insulin (with or without tablets),** you will be advised to test between one and four times a day (depending on how often you take your insulin doses), varying the times between just before and two hours after meals.

▶ **Testing patterns are individual.** Remember the whole point of testing is to measure the effects of your medication, food intake and physical activity. The amount you test will depend on your own personal situation and the results you are aiming for.

* Based on Diabetes UK Care Recommendation for Self Blood Glucose Monitoring.

Be part of a strong health-care team

Your usual GP may be the one helping you to manage your diabetes, but it takes a team of people to properly manage diabetes so that your feet, kidneys, eyes – even your diet and exercise – all receive care because diabetes affects your whole body.

If you're struggling with your blood glucose, consult a specialist. If your blood glucose readings aren't showing any improvement, even after following your doctor's advice closely for at least 12 to 16 weeks, ask your GP to refer you to a diabetes specialist nurse or doctor, also known as a diabetologist. This is a doctor who specialises in treating people with diabetes and you may be able to see them at your usual surgery or health centre. A diabetes specialist nurse will have a great deal of experience in helping people identify what might be contributing to variable blood glucose levels. He or she can also usually liaise with diabetes specialist doctors, dietitians and podiatrists, depending on your need. Importantly, the specialist will be able to offer you diabetes education courses where you can meet and share experiences with other people who may have coped with similar situations to yours and so may be able to help.

Make healthy eating habits a priority. What you eat and when you eat it affect your blood glucose more than any other lifestyle choice. If you have diabetes, you may need a personal eating plan tailored to your needs to help you to meet your blood glucose goals. The person who can help you form that plan is a registered dietitian who specialises in helping people with diabetes. The dietitian will help you to calculate how much food you should be eating, learn portion control, understand healthy food choices and plan meals that will fit your lifestyle. Not all registered dietitians specialise in diabetes, so make sure you are referred to one who does.

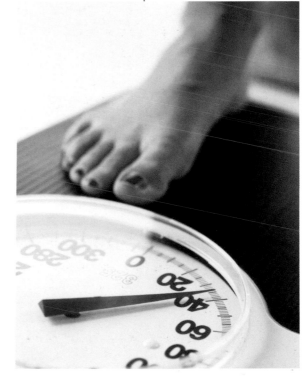

If you saw a dietitian or nutritionist years ago, it's time to see one again. Even if you've had diabetes for many years, it can be very helpful to see a nutritionist or dietitian to take stock of your current needs. Nutritional and calorie requirements change with age, and guidelines for eating with diabetes may also have changed since you

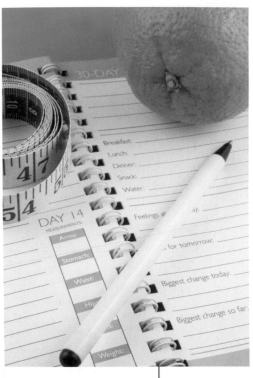

were diagnosed. A visit to a dietitian can also renew your motivation to eat better. You may even go home with some enjoyable new recipes to try.

Have the backs of your eyes checked at least once a year. Chronic high blood glucose can damage blood vessels in your retina (the inner layer of the eyes), which increases your risk of vision disorders and even blindness. You will be invited to have your eyes screened for retinopathy, which might be at a hospital clinic, with an optometrist or at a mobile unit. At the appointment, you may have drops put into your eyes to dilate your pupils, and the photograph takes seconds to complete. It may be possible for you to see the photograph immediately, but there is also a rigorous checking process to make sure the results are accurate. The screening photographer will be able to tell you about how you will receive the results.

See your dentist twice a year. As a child you learned that sugar causes tooth decay. Having high blood glucose can wreak havoc on your teeth, too. The bacteria which cause gum disease and cavities tend to proliferate when blood glucose isn't well controlled. That's why people with diabetes are more prone to gum disease, which is also linked to an increased risk of heart disease. See your dentist regularly, brush and floss daily, and be aware of any sores, tenderness or redness of your gums.

golden rule

Keep – and study – a food diary

Itemising each piece of food that passes your lips might seem like a pain, but it can do you some real good. It's easy to forget, or minimise, the snacking you did when you were making the lasagna for dinner, or the bite of blood-sugar-raising birthday cake you couldn't resist at the office party. Unconscious habits and patterns become more obvious when you see them in print. Plus, knowing that you'll be reviewing a food diary with your dietitian or diabetes specialist nurse might give you the willpower to refuse the cake and pick up an apple instead.

Take your feet to an expert. It's hard to imagine that a simple blister or cut could lead to foot amputation but, if the injury turns into an ulcer that becomes infected, it's all too possible. That's why it's so critical to take good care of your feet. A podiatrist is the member of the team who will check for any sores, blisters, bruises, cracks or cuts that are resistant to healing, as well as check for tingling or numbness in your feet. These health professionals can confirm nerve problems by doing a variety of tests using a tuning fork to see if you can detect vibrations, or by using heat or cold to see if you can detect these sensations. At your annual care planning appointment discuss with your doctor or practice nurse how often you should see or wish to see a podiatrist.

Four common diabetes tests

Here's a crib sheet on common tests you may be asked to have taken before or at your first clinic visit.

- **HbA1c:** This is a simple blood test done in a laboratory that shows your average blood glucose levels over approximately the last three months. The test is usually performed every three to six months to give you and your health professional more information about how well your diabetes treatment is working. The blood can be taken any time, regardless of what you've eaten. Typically, you want to see a number that is between 6.5% and 7.5%. If your levels are too high, you may need to alter your treatment plan to bring your blood glucose levels down.

- **Microalbuminuria:** This is a urine test, usually performed annually, that shows how well your kidneys are functioning by measuring albumin, a protein whose presence indicates early stage kidney damage at a time when it could be reversed or halted.

- **Creatinine:** This is a routine test of your kidney function. Creatinine is a waste product that is normally removed from the body by the kidneys, but if your kidneys are functioning less well, the level of creatinine in the blood increases.

- **Cholesterol and triglycerides:** This blood test, usually done annually, checks your levels of three kinds of fats. LDL, or 'bad' cholesterol, is a waxy fat that can build up and harden on the walls of your arteries. Levels should be under 2mmol/l. HDL, or 'good' cholesterol, is a healthy fat that actually removes the LDL from your veins and arteries. For people with diabetes, HDL should be above 1mmol/l. Triglycerides are the circulating storage form of fat, which your body produces from excess glucose or fat. Too much can cause hardening of the arteries. Your levels should be less than 1.7mmol/l.

golden rule

Get an annual flu vaccination

The effects of flu can be greater when you have diabetes because of the upset in your blood glucose levels that the illness can cause. This can sometimes lead to hospital admission. It's particularly serious if you are older or have complications of diabetes already. Diabetes UK recommends that all people with diabetes have an annual flu vaccination. The vaccination is available for free through your GP and takes only seconds. At the moment, not everyone who is offered the injection takes up the opportunity – so watch out for your invitation this winter.

When you visit your podiatrist, take the shoes you wear most often. The podiatrist can tell you whether your shoes are appropriate and whether you need any adjustments to your footwear, such as insoles or added padding.

Ask about local health walks or exercise on prescription. Many local areas offer health walks especially for people who would benefit from a bit more activity but in an enjoyable and sociable way. Anyone can join in and your clinic or surgery will have details. Also, your GP can refer you to your local leisure centre or gym for reduced-price, or even free, consultations with fitness trainers so that you can have a training programme designed specially for you. Taking up one of these opportunities might give you that extra push you need to help you to lose those stubborn pounds.

Speak to a counsellor. Mental health professionals such as psychologists or family therapists can offer additional support for dealing with the personal and emotional side of living with diabetes. Psychologists and family therapists will be able to offer individual or family therapy to help you to deal with the stress and depression that can often accompany a chronic disease.

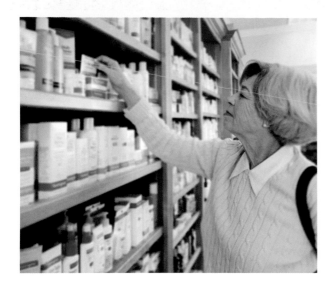

9

In the pharmacy

It's not just a place to pick up

prescriptions; you can come here for

other supplies, expert advice and

information about your medicines.

It all helps to give you better

control of your diabetes.

Get friendly with your pharmacist

Until now, your only interaction with your pharmacist may have been from afar, watching him or her counting capsules into bottles. But your pharmacist does far more than meets the eye. He or she can help you to understand your medication and give you useful information about new developments in diabetes treatment.

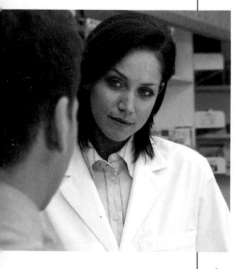

Shop at only one pharmacy. Having all your medication records in one place reduces your risk of taking duplicate medicines or experiencing dangerous drug interactions. You'll also feel more at ease asking questions or bringing up concerns if you're friendly with your local pharmacist.

Check your prescription while you're at the shop. Read the label and look at the pills or liquid as soon as you pick up your prescription – not when you get home – to make sure it's the right drug at the right dosage. If you're collecting a medication that you've taken before and it looks different, you will then have the chance to ask about it.

Ask for a meeting with your pharmacist to review your medicines. Many pharmacies are creating designated areas where you can talk to a pharmacist and have a medicines check or medicines use review. Call in or phone to make an appointment, and bring all your medications and any vitamins, herbal supplements and other over-the-counter items you take regularly. It's possible that you are taking two medications that do the same thing, or a medication that could be taken less often. After a medicines review by the pharmacist, you and your GP (or whoever prescribes your medicines) will be given a printout of what changes you have discussed and agreed so that this information is shared.

Take notes. Make a note of the answers to your questions or important points about new medications you're taking so you can review them at home, when you're under less pressure.

Have follow-up meetings with your pharmacist. Arrange to have a review whenever you are changing, adding to or reducing medications.

Devise a daily medications strategy. The more tablets and injections you have to take, the harder it is to remember every dose, especially when you take different ones at different times of day. Using a daily or weekly tablet organiser, leaving yourself a note by the kettle, or keeping a supply of tablets at work, might help to jog your memory. Devise a personal strategy that suits your daily routine.

Disclose any allergies or adverse reactions to drugs. Make sure that allergic reactions or bad side effects from any drugs you've taken in the past are still in your records. Be specific about what happened when you took them. Did you have a rash? Nausea? If you move and switch pharmacies, be sure to update your information.

Know who's who. Technicians help pharmacists by preparing medications, counting tablets and labelling bottles. Pharmacy assistants (the people you usually see behind the counter) are often cashiers who handle money and stock shelves. They can't necessarily answer your medication questions, but they will pass on your queries to the pharmacist.

Ask about diabetes or other health screening days. Increasingly, pharmacists are performing screening tests for diabetes, high blood pressure and cholesterol levels. While this might not be necessary for you, it might be useful to encourage family members to have checks, especially if Type 2 diabetes runs in your family. Screening tests are always personally supervised by the pharmacist and include a consultation about the possible meaning of the results and what to do next.

Talk to your pharmacist if you're feeling low. Sometimes diabetes, on top of everything else, can get you down and just talking can do a lot of good. Speaking to an experienced professional who is readily available is even better. Your pharmacist may know about a therapy or neighbourhood support group, plus other local treatments. It's no substitute for your GP or diabetes specialist, but it can help.

golden rule

Carry a list of all your medicines and supplements

This will be handy to have for consultations with doctors, pharmacists, dietitians and other health professionals. It could also prove helpful in the event of an emergency. Include supplements and over-the-counter remedies you take regularly. Next to the name of the medication or supplement, include the date of the prescription (where applicable), why you are taking it (what is it supposed to do?), the dosage and how many times a day you take it.

Obtaining diabetes supplies and equipment

Having diabetes isn't quite like having, say, high cholesterol. There's simply more equipment involved. And maybe we should be thankful it exists, because without blood-glucose meters, for instance, treating the disease would be much more difficult.

Now that there are more than 180 million people in the world who suffer from diabetes – and the numbers are rapidly increasing – it isn't surprising that many pharmacies are beginning to stock a wide range of diabetes equipment, so you might need a little help working your way through the various options.

Know what's on prescription and what's not. Your GP, practice nurse, diabetes specialist doctor or nurse will be able to prescribe for you the following items: all the tablets and insulin you need; insulin delivery devices such as pens; blood glucose monitoring strips and lancets; a sharps disposal container; some hypoglycaemia remedies such as glucose gel and glucagon injections. What you can't get on a normal prescription are: finger-pricking devices; blood glucose meters; insulin pumps and equipment; glucose tablets, drinks or other hypoglycaemia treatments. In certain circumstances, when agreed with your local health organisation, you may be able to obtain items such as an insulin pump and related supplies.

Do your homework before buying a blood glucose meter. There are many meters on the market and, although they are not very expensive, they all have different features and capacities.

golden rule

Test and clean your monitor regularly

If your monitor is old or dirty, if you've coded it wrongly, or if your test strips have expired or been exposed to heat or dampness, you'll get incorrect readings, which are worse than useless – they're misleading. Follow the manufacturer's instructions for how and when to clean the machine. To make sure you're getting accurate readings from your meter, use the quality control solution that comes with your meter, or order some from the manufacturer. This solution contains a fixed amount of glucose (the level is given on your test-strip pot). If your meter gives you a result in the suggested range, then it is giving you reliable blood test results, too.

Organisations such as Diabetes UK (www.diabetes.org.uk) have comparison information about all meters and all the contact details for the companies that manufacture them, so you can decide what's right for you before you buy one.

Decide on the features you want the most. Some meters require less blood than others and hold more readings than others. Some can talk you through the steps of taking and testing your blood. With others you can download results to your computer and even create charts to give you a picture of your glucose control at different times of the day over time. (If you buy this kind, make sure it will work with your home computer.) Work with your diabetes specialist nurse or practice nurse to decide which features are most important for you. Some people like lots of extra features; on the other hand, maybe a big display and ease of use are all you need.

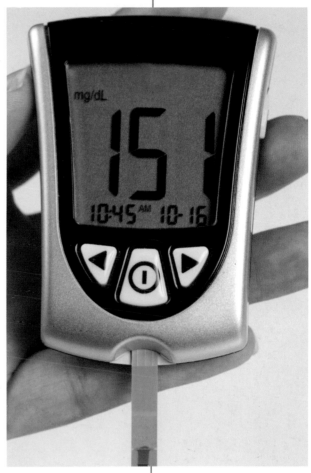

Buy a meter that doesn't require coding. Since test strips may vary from batch to batch, some meters require you to enter a code (found on the pot of test strips). This calibrates the meter to the batch of test strips. Other models have a 'no coding' feature. That's handy because forgetting to 'code' a meter is cited as one of the most frequent reasons that blood glucose is recorded inaccurately.

Use the logbook that comes with your meter. The only way to know how various foods or exercise affects your blood glucose is to check your levels often and write down the results. Most meters include a notebook for this purpose; you can also obtain them at your diabetes clinic. Don't stop at recording your results; sit down and examine them, looking for patterns. Bring your logbook every time you visit your doctor, dietitian and diabetes nurse. They can help you to make sense of the results.

Keep test strips cool and dry. The shelf life of test strips can be affected by heat and dampness. The bathroom is not a good place to store them.

Stock up on other useful items

The wonders you can find in an average pharmacy! Whether it's glucose tablets, a blood pressure machine, a healthy snack or good foot moisturiser, you can find all of these while you are waiting to pick up your prescription. Next time you are in your local pharmacy have a browse around the shelves to see what's on offer.

Buy a tablet organiser. Many people who have diabetes take eight to twelve different medications, vitamins and other supplements a day. Keeping track of that many pills is difficult, as is remembering which ones you have already taken, and what still needs to be swallowed. Pick up a tablet organiser that has flip-top compartments to contain all your tablets for each day of the week. You'll fill it up once a week and then be able to tell at a glance what you have and haven't taken. Your pharmacist will be able to advise you on the different types available.

Buy several bottles or packs of glucose. You'll find small and large bottles of glucose drinks and several varieties of glucose tablets on the pharmacy shelves. These products are made of glucose for treating low blood glucose. If you are particularly prone to low blood glucose episodes, it's a good idea to have several bottles or packets – one for the car, your desk at work, at home, and one packed in your suitcase when travelling. Throw a few tablets into a zip-close bag to carry in your handbag or pocket when you are going out for an evening, a family picnic or other outdoor event.

Consider a home blood pressure monitor. If you struggle with high blood pressure, tracking your levels at home can help you to keep track of your levels between clinic appointments and maybe even to lower those levels. Home tests may even provide truer results than a test at a clinic if you're one of those people who gets nervous

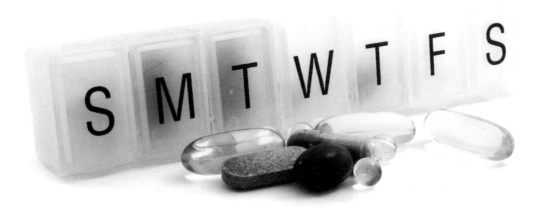

in a consultation room. It's easiest to use a fully automatic monitor and best to choose one with a cuff that measures your blood pressure at your upper arm, rather than at your wrist or finger, as these usually give the most accurate readings, advises the Blood Pressure Association. And make sure the monitor you choose has been 'clinically validated' for accuracy, meaning that it has been vigorously product-tested. (The association features a list of clinically validated monitors on its website at www.bpassoc.org.uk). Ask the pharmacist to tell you the cuff size you need for your arm as your readings will be wrong if the cuff size is incorrect. Always follow the manufacturer's instructions and make sure you can read the numbers on the monitor. Your monitor should be recalibrated every two years to ensure it continues to give accurate results; the manufacturer is likely to charge a fee for this service.

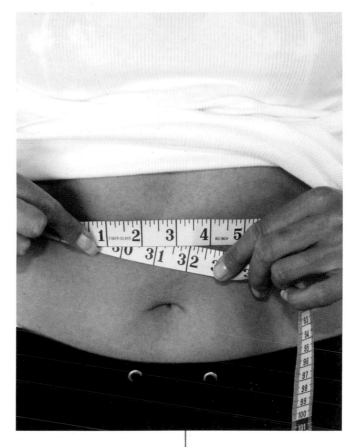

Ask your health professional if you should check your cholesterol at home. Most pharmacies now sell home cholesterol tests. Most are accurate, if you use them properly (many require you to fast, which people tend to forget to do). They can be useful if you're taking a cholesterol-lowering drug and want to see how well it, and your dietary changes, are working between clinic appointments. Look for a test that measures LDL ('bad') and HDL ('good') cholesterol in addition to total cholesterol. Some also measure triglycerides, blood fats associated with a higher risk of heart disease. Talk to your health professionals about the results and any changes you need to make.

Pick up a tape measure. It's one of the easiest ways to keep tabs on your heart health and to keep diabetes complications under control. Research shows that a waistline bigger than 88cm (34½in) for women and 102cm (40in) for men increases your risk of heart disease, high blood pressure and stroke. Measure your ankles, too; if they are swollen it's a sign that you are retaining water, and your doctor should be notified. Water retention is a side effect of some diabetes drugs.

>> continued on page 162

Herbs and supplements for diabetes

Pharmacies, health food shops and even supermarkets stock numerous kinds of vitamin and mineral supplements that claim to improve a whole range of conditions including diabetes. Although they have not been tested or regulated in the same way that drugs are, there are some clinical trials supporting their efficacy. Below are a selection of supplements that may be helpful, but do check with your GP or diabetes specialist nurse before taking them, to make sure they don't interact with your prescribed medicines.

Magnesium

Magnesium deficiency is not uncommon in people with diabetes, and it has been shown to affect blood glucose levels of people with Type 2 diabetes. Some studies suggest that supplementing with magnesium may improve insulin function and lower blood glucose levels, but other studies have shown no benefit. Ask your doctor if you can be tested for deficiency before supplementing with magnesium. Research suggests a single daily dose of 250-350mg.

Chromium

This trace mineral is thought to enhance the action of insulin as well as being involved in carbohydrate, fat and protein metabolism. Some research shows that it helps normalise blood glucose for people with Type 1 and Type 2 diabetes – but only in people who are deficient in chromium. So once again, it is worth checking that you are deficient before taking the supplement. Based on the research, a daily dose of 200mcg has been suggested.

Gamma-linolenic acid

Gamma-linolenic acid, or GLA, is a fatty acid found in evening primrose oil. Some research suggests that people with diabetes have lower than optimal levels of GLA, and studies have found that the supplement can reduce and prevent nerve pain associated with diabetes. The suggested daily dosage is 270-540mcg.

Alpha-lipoic acid

Called ALA for short, this potent antioxidant neutralises many types of free radicals. A build-up of free radicals, caused in part by high blood glucose, can lead to nerve damage and other problems. ALA may also help muscle cells take up blood glucose. In a German study, a team of scientists had 40 adults take either an ALA supplement or a placebo. At the end of the four-week study, the ALA group had improved their insulin sensitivity by 27 per cent. The placebo group showed no improvement. Other studies have shown a decrease in nerve pain, numbness and burning.

Research suggests that a daily dose of 600-800mcg can be effective.

B vitamins

Everyone needs B vitamins in their diet for healthy nerve functioning – and in people with diabetes it is perhaps even more important to ensure that you are getting all your B vitamins. The B vitamins work together so it is best to take a B complex such as Brewer's yeast, or other formulation that contains the major B vitamins. Biotin, B_6 and B_{12} are particularly relevant for people with diabetes, as they may have low levels of biotin, which is needed by the body to utilise glucose. Boosting levels may therefore help lower blood glucose in Type 1 and Type 2 diabetes. Vitamins B_6 and B_{12} are thought to help with the repair of nerve damage associated with diabetes.

Vitamin C

Because vitamin C is a water-souble vitamin and is not stored in the body, it is worth considering taking a supplement to make sure you are getting sufficient. It has been suggested that increased levels of vitamin C in the bloodstream can lower the levels of sorbitol – a harmful sugar that in high enough concentrations can lead to complications of diabetes such as retinopathy. The usual dose is around 1-3g daily.

Balanced diet best

Though supplements can seem to be a magic bullet, the truth – acknowledged by most medical specialists – is that nothing beats a healthy, balanced diet for all-round health and vitality. A diet that includes at least five portions a day of fruit and vegetables, whole grains, a good mix of lean protein such as chicken and pulses, two servings a week of an oily fish such as mackerel, plus nuts and seeds should provide you with all the vitamins and minerals that you need. Shop-bought supplements do not come cheap – so you can save yourself some money by simply tuning up your diet (see Chapter 1).

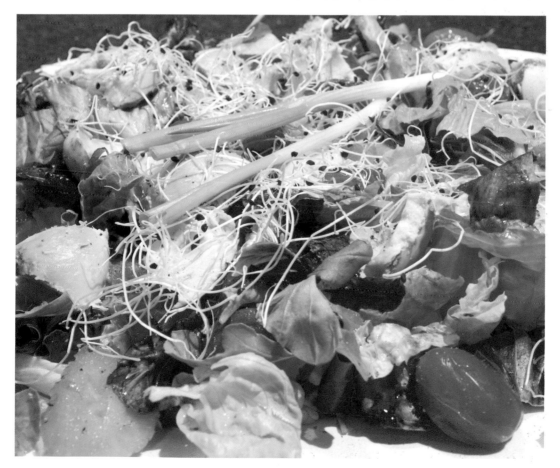

Keep feet happy with seam-free socks. Your pharmacy may stock socks for people with nerve damage or loss of sensation in their feet. These socks fit comfortably, but not too tightly, and they don't have any seams that could cause sore spots or blisters. People with loss of sensation in their feet may not notice chafing from ordinary socks, and chafing could lead to blisters and infection.

Pick up a healthy lunch or snack. Many pharmacies sell a range of food and drinks, including low-calorie, low-fat options and easy-to-eat portions of fruit and vegetables. If you're someone who's often caught on the hop at mealtimes, you might want to keep a supply for emergencies. The carbohydrates they contain are digested slowly to help keep blood glucose levels steady. They are useful to keep hunger at bay when you are shopping during your lunch hour. They are also good to have to hand when the tempting cake trolley comes round the office in the afternoon.

Buy – and use – a good moisturiser. High blood glucose can contribute to dry skin, which in turn can lead to cracks that can lead to infection – and then you're in trouble. So make a commitment to use a moisturiser every day or night. While you might see special moisturisers labelled for people with diabetes, don't feel limited to these, which often cost more. Any moisturiser that's thick enough to stay put and that doesn't irritate your skin will do.

Don't use deodorant soaps. These tend to be drying and irritating to the skin, and dry, irritated skin is more likely to crack and become vulnerable to infection. It is better to choose moisturising soaps instead.

Look for sugar-free over-the-counter medicines. Your blood glucose may already be on the high side when you're unwell, so why get unnecessary sugar from cold and cough remedies? While the sugar in these won't affect your blood glucose much, neither will it hurt to look for or ask your pharmacist about sugar-free versions of cough syrups, lozenges, chewable painkillers and decongestants.

Buy the most protective sunscreen. Certain diabetes drugs and blood-pressure drugs make the skin more sensitive to the sun, so it's especially important that you protect yourself. A bad sunburn can even raise your blood glucose and may take longer to heal than for someone without diabetes. Choose a sunscreen that has at least an SPF of 15 and look for a 'broad-spectrum' brand that protects against both UVA and UVB light. Use plenty of sunscreen on all areas of exposed skin and apply it at least half an hour before heading out into the sun to give your skin a chance to absorb it. Reapply every 2 hours.

golden rule

Set the timer when you brush your teeth

Dentists recommend brushing for 2 to 3 minutes to get teeth clean, but most of us spend far less time than that caring for our pearly whites. Set a timer and you'll realise just how long 3 minutes really is. Brushing thoroughly is especially important for people with diabetes, who are at increased risk of gum disease.

Throw out old sunscreen. If you've had a bottle that's been lying around for several years or has been living in the glove compartment of a hot car, buy a new bottle – the old one has undoubtedly lost strength and will no longer be effective.

Stock up on dental-care items. Because people with diabetes are more susceptible to gum disease, good oral hygiene is essential. Make sure you have plenty of floss and check with your dentist for the best type to use – especially if you have bridges. You can also buy small disposable brushes that help you to clean between your teeth. Fluoride toothpaste will help to protect your teeth and your dentist may also recommend an anti-bacterial oral mouthwash.

Replace your toothbrush every three months. If the bristles are frayed or bent outwards, replace more frequently. Otherwise, your brush won't get your teeth clean, and you'll be transferring a lot of bacteria to your mouth. Look for a brush with soft bristles so you don't bruise your gums, and while you're in the toothbrush aisle, pick up some floss, too – then use it.

Consider buying an electric toothbrush. Studies show that they remove plaque better than manual toothbrushes and some models now have a built-in 2 minute timer.

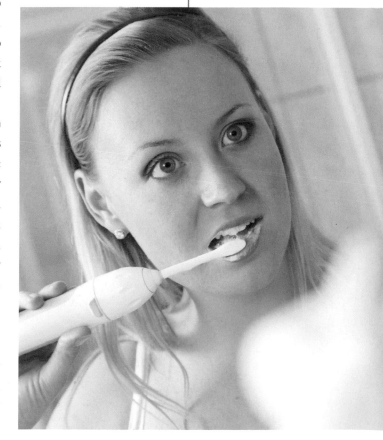

How to choose vitamins and more

Some doctors may suggests a daily multivitamin to ensure that you get your full complement of essential nutrients, but the shelves are lined with choices. Which should you pick? Do you need more than one type? The advice below will help you to choose, but be sure to check with your doctor before taking any new supplement.

Talk to your dietitian before buying. It's a good idea to discuss your potential vitamin needs with a registered dietitian. Once the specialist has a good idea of your eating habits and has run blood tests to check for deficiencies, he or she may be able to suggest any vitamins you might need. A once-a-day vitamin can be useful, or your nutritionist might recommend some extra supplements based on your needs. Ask him or her to write down all the recommendations and dosages.

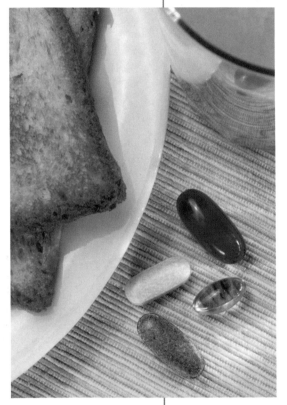

Be wary of health-food shop 'experts'. It's unlikely that these people are registered dietitians or certified health professionals of any sort. Check any recommendations with your own dietitian before you buy.

Check the RDA values on your multivitamin. It's best to get most of your vitamins and minerals from a healthy diet, but a good multivitamin may be suggested to supplement nutrient deficiencies. European Union regulations require Recommended Daily Amounts to be shown on food and supplement labels. To get the best value for money, find a multivitamin that gives a high percentage of the RDA for a good proportion of its components. But it is not imperative that a multivitamin gives you 100 per cent as you will be getting vitamins and minerals from your food.

Beware of other inflated claims. Before you waste money on a formula that promises better immune health or boasts super-high levels of antioxidants, talk to your registered dietitian. It's probably better to focus on eating a diet full of vegetables and fruits than to seek a few extra ingredients in a multivitamin.

Take vitamins with a meal. Some vitamins and supplements can cause nausea if you take them on an empty stomach, so take them with a meal. Some people find it easier to remember if they get in the habit of doing so routinely with breakfast, lunch or dinner.

Ask your doctor about iron. Many multivitamins contain iron, but men and postmenopausal women don't usually need more of this mineral than they get from food, so ask your doctor whether or not you should choose a formulation that contains it. Too much iron can cause toxic effects, not to mention constipation. If you are concerned that your iron levels may be low (for instance, if you are a strict vegetarian), ask your doctor for a blood test to check your iron levels.

If you're a woman, consider taking calcium supplements. A lack of calcium and vitamin D leads to an increased risk of developing diabetes. If you already have diabetes, these supplements can still be useful because they will help to protect your bones; this is important because older people with diabetes are more susceptible to bone fractures and osteoporosis. Calcium also helps your body with contractions of muscles and blood vessels. Research suggests doses of 1,000mg a day, or 1,200mg a day if you're over 50. Take it in split doses of half in the morning and evening; the body can't absorb higher doses. Men should check with their doctors before supplementing with calcium.

Calcium supplements containing vitamin D may be best. Experts are learning more and more about the important roles vitamin D plays in the body. For instance, low levels are associated with increased insulin resistance and decreased insulin secretion, and also heart disease and stroke. Obese people are at higher risk of vitamin D

Should you take antioxidants?

Research suggests that people with diabetes may need more of certain antioxidants, such as vitamins C and E, and that antioxidants play a role in preventing diabetes complications such as nerve damage and eye problems. One study even found that supplementing with vitamin E (400 IU), vitamin C (500–1000mg), magnesium (300–600mg) and zinc (30mg) daily for three months significantly lowered blood glucose in a test group. But other studies on antioxidant supplements have yielded mixed results, and supplements aren't without dangers. Too much magnesium, for instance, can potentially be harmful in people with decreased kidney function. And a study that looked at the mineral selenium and its effect on skin cancer revealed that the supplement increased the risk of diabetes by nearly 50 per cent.

Much more research is under way, but for now, most experts advise getting the bulk of your antioxidants from a diet rich in fruit, vegetables and beans, and filling any gaps with a basic multivitamin.

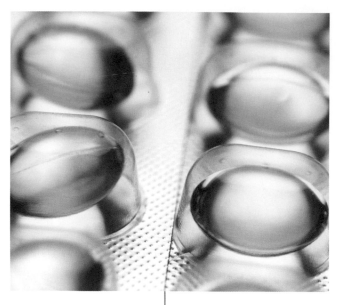

deficiency, and the deficiency appears to predispose people to become obese. Research suggests that vitamin D may also help to protect against cancer.

Ask your doctor or pharmacist about fish oil capsules. Many studies show that taking fish oil can lower the risk of heart attack and stroke risk by lowering triglyceride levels, helping to prevent dangerous blood clots and more. That's good news for people with diabetes, who are at an increased risk of both conditions. Fish oil also combats low-grade inflammation in the body, which contributes to diabetes and other chronic diseases. But fish oil supplements aren't for everyone, so seek advice from your doctor. Taking the supplements with food can help reduce the burping often associated with fish oils, as can choosing a fish-oil supplement that contains citrus essence. A typical dosage is 1–3g daily, but don't exceed 3g, as an excessive intake may raise harmful LDL cholesterol.

And should you be taking a daily low-dose aspirin? Heart disease is a major risk for people who suffer from diabetes. Getting plenty of exercise, reaching and maintaining your optimum weight, and eating healthily all help. But Diabetes UK currently recommends that people diagnosed with diabetes, aged 50 or over, in the groups below, should be offered low-dose aspirin treatment as well – though you should always consult your GP first as new research is constantly being published.

* Who have had diabetes for more than 10 years
* Who are already having treatment for high blood pressure
* Who have diabetic retinopathy or nerve damage
* Who are of South Asian or Black African Caribbean origin
* Who smoke
* Who have a family history of heart disease

Daily aspirin should not be taken if you have gastric or duodenal ulcers, aspirin allergy, a tendency to bleed, a past history of gastro-intestinal bleeding, active hepatic (liver) disease, a history of asthma or have ever suffered asthma as a result of taking aspirin, uncontrolled high blood pressure, or if you are currently being treated with an anticoagulant such as Warfarin.

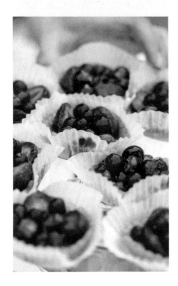

10

At the restaurant

Who doesn't love dining out?

But when you go to a restaurant,

try to eat healthily – just as you

would at home. Then the price

you pay will only be the bill

and not your health.

Get set – before you sit down

Low lighting, soft music, attentive waiters and mouthwatering aromas wafting from the kitchen: restaurants are in the business of making you feel like a VIP. Because the longer you stay, the more relaxed you feel, and the more money the restaurant makes, as you forget about how much you're eating and spending. The best way not to overindulge is to step through the door prepared.

Sneak an advance peek at the menu. To help ensure that the atmosphere does not dissolve your determination to eat well, do a little reconnaissance before you even leave the house. Look online for the menus of the restaurant or restaurant chain; some chains even post nutritional information. Look for options that fit into your eating plan and identify dishes that you know you must stay away from.

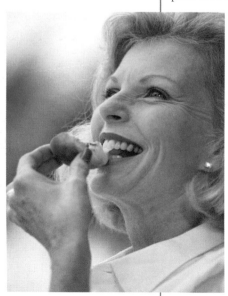

Scan the menu for healthy options. Many people these days are trying to make healthy choices when they dine out, and restaurants are beginning to take notice. Most now offer plenty of salads and other no-frills healthy dishes on their menus where meats are baked or grilled, and vegetables are usually steamed. If you're counting calories and fat, head straight for the healthy options on the menu.

Have a healthy snack at home an hour before your restaurant reservation. That's assuming that you're eating an hour later than you normally do, as people tend to do when they eat out. (If you're eating at the normal time and you didn't have an afternoon snack planned, skip it.) Munch on a small piece of fruit and 25g of low-fat cheese, or a couple of pieces of celery slathered with a tablespoon of peanut or cashew butter. Not only will a snack curb your appetite, but the feeling of having just eaten will keep you from mindlessly picking at the prawn crackers or complimentary breadsticks.

Before you go out, prepare a healthy, home-made dessert. Make a light berry crumble, a sugar-free jelly with fresh fruit, or a baked apple sprinkled with cinnamon and sugar substitute. Later, at the restaurant when you're handed the dessert menu – or even worse, when a waiter brings over a tray of fatty, sugary confections – you'll remember that you have a delicious treat waiting for you at home.

Wear a tight skirt or close-fitting trousers. Whether you dine at a four-star restaurant or not, what you wear can affect what your order. With a tight-waisted skirt or trousers tugging at your tummy, you literally won't have room to gorge on a big dinner. And the chances are, if you're also wearing your favourite blouse or best shirt, you'll be afraid of ruining it, which might deter you from eating very fatty meals or rich sauces. The worst thing to wear? Loose or elasticated trousers with plenty of room for expansion.

In the car park, pop a piece of gum into your mouth. Just as brushing your teeth early in the evening keeps you from late-night snacking, popping some mint chewing gum into your mouth just before you go into the restaurant can help you to avoid sugary soft drinks and tempting appetisers. Only after the waiter takes your order should you discreetly remove the gum; that still gives you at least 15 minutes for the minty taste to diminish and for your mouth to return to normal so that your meal tastes as enjoyable as you'd hoped.

whip it together!

Ambrosia

This treat, under 150kcal, tastes best after it's chilled in the fridge for a few hours, making it the perfect 'nightcap' dessert after a dinner out.

Cut a small **pineapple** into 2cm chunks (or use about 400g canned pineapple) and cut 2 large **bananas** into ½cm thick slices. Toss both into a Pyrex bowl. Peel and segment three **navel oranges** over the bowl, allowing the juice from the oranges to coat the fruit. Gently fold in 25g miniature **marshmallows** and 2 tablespoons

desiccated **coconut.** Cover with cling film and refrigerate for at least 2 hours. Before serving, garnish with fresh **mint** sprigs.

Serves 6.

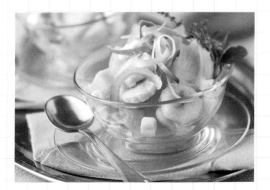

Clever dining-out strategies

A generation ago, restaurant meals were reserved for special occasions. Now we eat out so often that we don't even bother to get dressed up – and sometimes, we even opt for a takeaway because we can't be bothered to sit down and be served. Why not step back into the past, and inject a little excitement and sense of occasion into restaurant outings? Whether you realise it or not, little decisions like where you should dine, with whom you eat, and what you do after you dine can all help you to control your diabetes.

Splash out on a fancy restaurant. Look for a restaurant that prides itself on using seasonal, local ingredients. Such places tend to serve smaller portions of top-quality foods, rather than gargantuan platters of inexpensive oily pastas and pizzas. How do you know if the ingredients are local? The menu will often mention the source of top-quality fish, meat or produce. If a chef has gone to the trouble and expense of acquiring, say, local wild salmon, he or she will want you to know how special it is and will prepare the fish in a way that will emphasise its quality. So it probably won't be fried or hidden under heavy sauces and that means fewer grams of fat and calories for you.

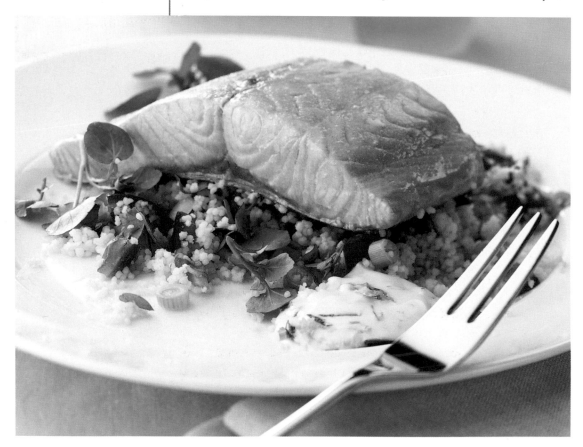

Dine with other health-conscious people. Research shows that diners tend to mimic the people around them. That means that if your friends order grilled fish and salads with the dressing on the side, you're more likely to do so, as well. Sample all the dishes when they're served. The variety will make you feel as if you've indulged more than you really have and you'll know what to order next time.

Frequent the same restaurants again and again. If you dine out often, this advice is for you. The more new choices you're faced with, the more easily you'll be seduced by foods you probably should not be eating. So you might be best advised to find a favourite restaurant and choose it whenever you can. Then you will limit temptation by ordering from the same old menu and choosing dishes you know work well for your blood glucose.

Plan one truly sinful meal out twice a year. You've been dreaming of that triple brownie sundae and home-made pasta at the local Italian restaurant since your last anniversary dinner there. So go! Always saying 'no' to food treats can make you resent your healthy diet. And even some nutritionists confess that they go out and have their 'weakness' food – maybe it's onion rings, chips or ice cream – once every six or eight months. To get maximum enjoyment from your special meal, make a reservation a month or two in advance. The further in advance your event is planned, the more pleasure you'll get when you finally dig in.

Save the gossip for your post-meal walk. Even a casual lunch with an old friend can turn into an exercise opportunity if you take an energised turn or two around a nearby park or the shopping centre afterwards. Light exercise is a sure way to help level your blood glucose if a meal has caused it to rise.

Check your blood glucose two hours after your meal. If the result is within your target range, you'll know to order the same thing when you go back. If it's not, avoid those dishes next time, or try to make adjustments to your meal, such as declining the bread or substituting a vegetable for the rice or potato.

golden rule

Save restaurant meals for special occasions

Several studies have found that the more people eat out, the more likely they are to be obese, and extra weight can make your insulin resistance worse – and your blood glucose harder to control. In one study, researchers followed more than 3,000 adults for 15 years, keeping track of their body weight, changes in insulin resistance, and how often they ate at fast-food restaurants. They found that people who ate fast food more than twice a week gained an average of 4.5kg more over 15 years than people who ate fast food less than once a week. Frequent fast-food eaters also had double the risk of becoming insulin resistant.

At the table

If you go to a party, you want to have a good time. So when you sit down at a restaurant table, be equally determined to eat well – and have fun. Focus on soaking up the atmosphere, relaxing with your partner or friends and enjoying the occasion and also, of course, the food – but in moderation.

Ask the waiter not to bring bread. You're likely to get plenty of starch in your meal (from your rice, potatoes and starchy vegetables), so save your carbohydrates for later.

After you've been seated, take a quick stroll around the dining room. Before you order, excuse yourself to wash your hands, and take the long route to the cloakroom. On your way there and back to your table, take a good look at other diners' dishes. This reconnaissance mission can be more useful for deciding what to order than the most well-meaning waiter. For a start, you'll see how big the restaurant's portions are, how good tonight's specials look, and whether the vegetable side dishes look fresh and healthy or are swimming in butter. When you get back to your seat, you'll be one of the best informed diners in the room.

Order a mixed salad to start. A small mixed salad usually contains two servings of vegetables and about 5g of fibre. Because of that fibre, salads are surprisingly filling. In fact, a study published in the *Journal of the American Dietetic Association* found that women who ate 100kcal salads before their main meals consumed about 12 per cent fewer calories during the meal. Just stick to vegetables in the salad, rather than fatty meats, cheeses and nuts.

Dress your own salad. It's true: a tasty dressing can absolutely make a salad. The problem is, chefs know this, too, and can be heavy-handed with their dressings. A typical restaurant Caesar salad is tossed with 65g of dressing, which adds about 360kcal and 38g of fat to otherwise healthy and very low-calorie Romaine lettuce. Ordering the same dressing on the side and topping your salad with just a tablespoon would add 77kcal and 8g of fat.

golden rule

Eat no more than you would at home

It's not at all unusual for a restaurant meal to contain more than half a day's worth of calories and fat. Eating a mega-sized portion can not only wreak havoc with your blood glucose, it could cause you to overeat for the next two days. When researchers studied the eating habits of 32 people, they found that when the subjects ate 50 per cent more at a meal, they continued to eat 16 per cent more calories for two days compared to when they ate a normal-sized meal. When their portion sizes doubled, they ate 26 per cent more calories for two days.

Start your meal with a clear soup. This is another proven strategy to take the edge off your hunger and help you to eat less of the main meal. In one study, people who ate a broth-based vegetable soup before lunch ended up consuming, on average, 20 per cent fewer calories overall. Avoid cheesy or creamy soups, such as French onion, broccoli and cheese, or vichyssoise.

Think for yourself when you order. Some restaurants hire consultants to tell them where to put what on the menu and how to price it – and it's money, not health, that they're after. For instance, they'll typically place dishes that they want you to buy just above the centre of the menu's first right-hand page. The two top and bottom dishes on a list are also the ones that diners tend to remember best, so restaurant owners tend to put the most expensive items in those places. The specialties (which also tend to be more expensive) might appear in big type, and cheaper meals in small type.

Speak up and ask for small changes to your dish. Don't be shy; most restaurants are happy to oblige, within reason. Just make your requests simple. If the item you have your eye on is fried, ask if it could be grilled instead. If it's coated in a buttery sauce, ask if the sauce can be left off. And remember that chefs aren't miracle workers. If you're tempted to make an unreasonable request, like asking for macaroni and cheese without the cheese, order something else.

Befriend the waiting staff. If whoever serves you has gone out of his or her way to ask the chef to grill your meat, steam your vegetables and put your sauce on the side, make a point of learning the person's name. Say thank you and leave a generous tip. The next time you're in the restaurant, ask to be seated in the same section. Eventually he or she will automatically do the things that you always ask for, like bringing you one piece of bread – preferably wholemeal. Restaurant regulars who are kind and generous to staff are always taken care of. (Staff talk to each other about their customers, so you're likely to get good service even if you're seated in another section.)

Have a starter and a salad instead of a main course. Many restaurants' main courses are at least twice as big as a standard serving. If you don't think you have the willpower to order a main course and not eat the whole thing, order a starter-sized dish instead. Healthy options include prawn cocktail, steamed mussels, hummus and pitta bread, and grilled chicken skewers (with sauce on the side). Ask the waiter to bring you one of these as your main dish, and dig into a salad when everyone else is eating their starters.

Substitute a side dish of broccoli instead of chips. Want to order the beefburger platter but don't want to be tempted by the French fries? Ask to substitute the restaurant's vegetable of the day for the fries. A serving of cooked broccoli, for example, contains no fat and just 27kcal – less than one-tenth the calories in a small order of French fries. Making the easy switch from chips to broccoli also saves you 3g of saturated fat and infuses your meal with about 80 per cent of your daily allowance of vitamin C.

Beware of the buffet. If the restaurant boasts all-you-can-eat platters and buffets, steer clear, however much a bargain it appears to be. One study found that when people served themselves food, as they do at buffets, they often gave themselves at least 25 per cent more food than a healthy portion. All-you-can-eat platters are just as bad – maybe worse – because the plate portion may look reasonable, but you quickly lose count of how many full plates you've been served.

Fix your gaze on a visual reminder. Cauliflower in cheese sauce, roast potatoes and roast pork with its crackling sounds great, but there's more saturated fat on that plate than you should eat in two days. It's at moments like this that you'll be glad you have a secret weapon in your handbag or wallet. Perhaps it's a photo of you a few years ago, looking very happy and a stone lighter. Your visual aid might even be a list of health goals you want to achieve – anything that will persuade you to make a healthier choice.

Avoid food drenched in rich sauces. Meat, fish, pasta or even vegetables that are bathed in a cream or cheese-based sauce can double the calories in the dish and add artery-clogging saturated fat. A standard serving of carbonara, for instance, contains about 25g of saturated fat – more than the 15g a heart-healthy 2,000kcal diet allows in an entire day. Bearing in mind that restaurants' portions can be double a normal 'serving', you could be consuming four to six times your daily allowance of saturated fat in one sitting.

Learn restaurant code words for 'very high in fat'. It's common for restaurants to make their food sound healthier and more fancy than it really is. One trick is to disguise dishes that are deep-fried. Anything that's called 'golden' or 'crispy' is probably deep-fried and should be avoided. Other words to look out for include 'au gratin', 'cheesy', 'creamy' and 'béarnaise', all of which are loaded with cheese, cream and/or butter.

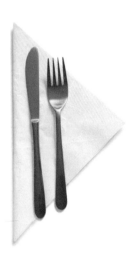

PLUS POINT
Try to avoid cream or cheese-based sauces; they can double the number of calories in a dish.

golden rule

Order your meat or fish grilled or baked

Dishes that are grilled or baked will almost always be lower in fat than those that are fried or sautéed. An order of fried chicken nuggets can contain as many as 23g of saturated fat, while a piece of grilled chicken or fish may only have 2g or 3g. Keeping your intake of saturated fat low – those following a 2,000kcal diet should eat a maximum of 15g of saturated fat per day – is crucial for people with diabetes. Saturated fat contributes to insulin resistance, which makes controlling your blood glucose more difficult; saturated fat also increases your risk of heart disease.

Look for dishes that are poached or slow-cooked rather than fried. Technically speaking, fried foods should be cooked on high heat with a small amount of fat, but restaurants are heavy-handed with butter and oil because they make food taste better. Tossing in an extra spoonful of oil can add as many as 11g of fat to your meal. Instead, ask for dishes where your meat is cooked in stock or wine, with minimal added fats. (The wine will burn off during cooking while the flavour remains.)

Ask for your vegetables steamed, not sautéed. Like all fried dishes, sautéed vegetables are often coated with more butter or oil than you need.

Order 'Cajun' chicken. 'Cajun' means that the meat has been coated in Cajun seasoning and thrown into a red-hot cast-iron skillet. Cajun seasoning blends cayenne pepper, black pepper, and onion and garlic powders, so it's quite delicious and also delivers a little kick. Cajun seasoning is one great way to get plenty of flavour without sauces, oils or other added calories.

Splash out on lobster but leave out the melted butter. Lobster – undoubtedly a luxury – can also be an extremely healthy choice: it contains only a few grams of fat, little carbohydrate and only a few hundred calories, according to size. The real danger lies in the dish of melted butter that comes with it. The simple act of squeezing lemon juice over your lobster rather than drowning it in 4 tablespoons of melted butter will save you an incredible 400kcal – probably about the same number of calories you eat for lunch – as well as 28g of saturated fat.

Controlling your portion size

The restaurant business is highly competitive; about 60 per cent of restaurants fail within their first three years. So they have to find a way to get you in and keep you coming back. As one restaurant consultant, Thomas J. Haas, puts it, 'The customer's perception of value should always come first' – and what most diners perceive as 'good value' is a lot of food for not a lot of money. If you rid yourself of that notion, your body will go home happy.

Share a main course. Most meals are large enough to split, so don't be afraid to share a main course. Just order an extra side salad and extra vegetables if you like. You'll save money, too.

Ask for a smaller portion. If you see mountains of food being served to other customers in the restaurant, ask whether you can have a half-portion. Most restaurants will be happy to oblige. Some restaurants feature 'light bites', which tend to be smaller versions of main courses – and you can even order something from the children's menu. You will save yourself money as well as unwanted calories, as research shows that people tend to eat what's on their plate.

At steak houses, order by weight. Unlike just about any other type of restaurant, steakhouses are specific about the weight of their portions – the Aberdeen Angus chain, for instance, boasts seven cuts of steak in various weights. This is both good and bad news for customers watching their portion sizes: good news because you know how much meat you're getting, but bad news because even the smallest portion will be bigger than the recommended 75g or 100g. Pick the smallest boneless (so the weight of the bone is not factored in) steak on the menu – or share a steak with your dining companion.

Visualise proper portion sizes. Then compare them to what's on your plate. If you've practised portion

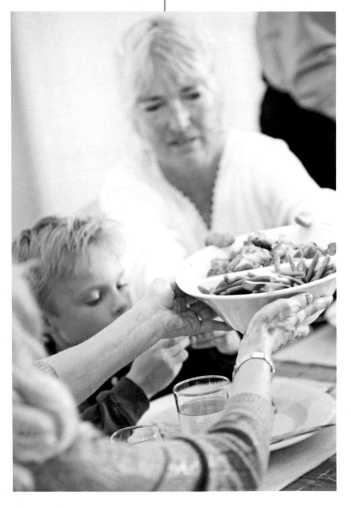

control at home, it should be just as easy to do at a restaurant. A serving of meat (about 75g) should be the size of a deck of cards, and a serving of pasta is 75g as a side dish (about half the size of a cricket ball), and twice that if it's your main course. If your meal arrives and your meat takes up half the plate, you'll know to cut it in half and take the rest home or give it to a friend who's dining with you.

Be on your best behaviour, and you'll eat less. Whether you're dining in a pub or at a four-star restaurant, you can actually consume less if you're perfectly behaved. For example, wait until everyone in your party has arrived, ordered and received their food before you dig into your starters. Keep your mouth busy by making polite conversation with everyone at the table, rather than stuffing your face while you listen. Put your fork down after every bite or two, and dab your lips with a napkin, or take a sip of water. Chew your food thoroughly before speaking. Those polite pauses can help you to slow down your eating.

Stay away from your 'downfall' foods. You know your own weaknesses. If you can't possibly stop at a healthy 75g portion of pasta, don't think about ordering it. If you tend to go overboard on the meat, order fish or a big salad. In a two-week study of 48 women with a history of bingeing, researchers found that half of their binges occurred in restaurants, nearly half happened at dinner, and more than half occurred at the weekends. Common binge foods included bread or pasta, sweets, high-fat meat and salty snacks.

Leave three bites of food on your plate. If you're in the habit of clearing your plate at every meal only to feel indigestion later on, you're learning the hard way that it takes 20 to 30 minutes for your brain to register that you're 100 per cent full. How much you can eat to feel pleasingly satisfied varies by individual; tonight, leave a few bites on your plate and see how you feel after your meal. Still full? Tomorrow night leave a few more bites on the plate, and so on. In time you will be able to put less on your plate to start with and you'll probably be surprised by how much more lively and less sluggish you feel after your restaurant meal.

If you order dessert, order only one for the table. Ask for spoons or forks for everyone. One bite that you savour can satisfy your craving and save you lots of calories and carbohydrates.

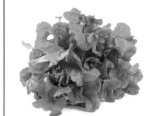

PLUS POINT
Ordering fish or a big salad will save you from yourself if you tend to go overboard on meat.

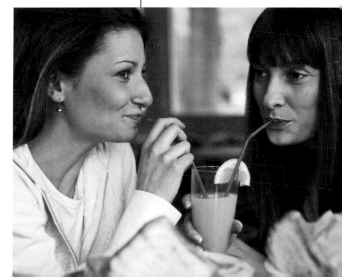

Drinking and dining

Alcohol has different effects on people with diabetes than it does on other people. It can cause low blood glucose for one thing. The good news is that light to moderate alcohol intake (a maximum of two units a day for women and three for men) is associated with a lower risk of dying of heart disease. Follow these guidelines, and a pint of beer or a glass of wine can be part of your dining experience.

Have a glass of wine or beer only if your blood glucose typically falls within your target range. If you check your blood glucose regularly, experts say that it's fine for both men and women to order up to two drinks at dinner. But if your levels are more erratic, try not to drink alcohol as it could cause you to experience hypoglycaemia and will make it more difficult for you to get your blood glucose into your target range.

Do not have an aperitif. Drinking alcohol before dinner is not a good idea, particularly for those who take insulin or other diabetes medications. Without food in your stomach, your blood glucose levels might already be low. Drink your alcohol with your food – or better still, at the end of the meal – to lessen your chances of developing hypoglycaemia.

Watch out for high-calorie cocktails. Some cocktails such as Pina Colada and other creamy concoctions contain as much as 280kcal. Go for lower calorie choices such as Bloody Mary or Martini as these have only 90kcal and very few carbohydrates.

Decide whether you want wine or dessert. It's easy to forget that drinks contain calories, just as solid foods do. If your blood glucose levels are within a healthy range, it's fine to indulge in a glass of wine with dinner, but you'll need to modify your food intake. A 150ml glass of wine contains about 120kcal, for example – two glasses contain roughly the same amount of calories as a 5cm square brownie.

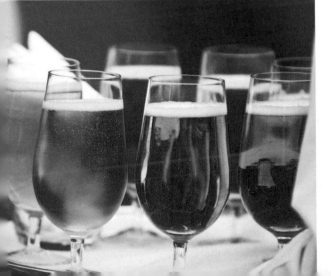

If you're counting calories, you'll need to plan ahead and decide whether a drink or a sweet treat is more appealing. If you are on insulin, you can't substitute alcohol for the carbohydrate-filled dessert. Your insulin dose is based on the amount of carbohydrates you eat. Alcohol has calories but you don't need insulin to cover it.

Don't confuse low blood glucose with being drunk. Sometimes slurred speech or difficulty speaking occurs with hypoglycaemia; this could be confused with being drunk.

Food to enjoy at Chinese and Thai restaurants

The good news about dining out at Chinese and Thai restaurants is that both cultures' foods really allow vegetables to shine – you're more likely to find a wide array of vegetarian dishes at these eateries than you are at almost any other type of restaurant. Protein-rich tofu, too, is plentiful, while butter and cream sauces are almost unheard of. The bad news is that Chinese and Thai dishes can be clogged with salt, sugar and calorie-heavy oils; it's not uncommon for a single Chinese dish to contain an entire day's worth of salt. The coconut milk in an average portion of a zesty Thai curry contains more than a day's worth of saturated fat.

Fill your teacup. Whether the restaurant serves green or black tea, have some. Tea is one of nature's most potent sources of anti-oxidants, and these free-radical scavengers help protect the body from the ravages of blood glucose, such as artery and nerve damage. Best of all, tea is calorie free.

Eat with chopsticks. It's easy to shovel in big mouthfuls of food with a fork. With chopsticks, each vegetable or slice of beef has to be picked up carefully and put safely into your mouth. Because of the skill and pace involved, the odds are you'll eat more slowly with chopsticks than with a fork. Another plus point is that when you eat with chopsticks, you're more likely to leave some of the fatty sauce behind on the plate.

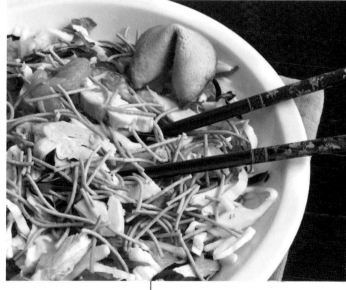

Avoid sweet-and-sour sauces. These sauces, which often come with lemon chicken or crispy beef, spell double trouble for the unwary diner. Not only are they high in sugar, but they also traditionally coat meats that have been battered and deep fried.

Order garlic or brown sauce, on the side. These contain less sugar than sweet-and-sour sauces, and they often come with stir-fried meat and vegetable dishes. They're typically sky-high in salt, though, so ask for them on the side and use sparingly.

Order prawn rather than beef. The US Center for Science in the Public Interest conducted a nutritional analysis of Chinese food and found that some of the healthiest choices (in terms of calories and fat) were prawn dishes. But you will need to ask for the sauce on the side, to keep the salt down.

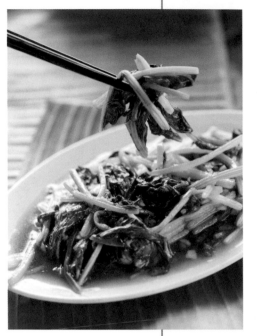

Limit your portions of rice. It can be easy to overdo it with rice. A typical takeaway serving of rice, for example, contains around 100g of carbohydrate (that's the same as 6 slices of bread). Aim to fill up on vegetable dishes and try to limit yourself to no more than half a serving (50g of carbohydrate) of rice (brown rice, if you can get it). To cut down on the fat content of your meal, always choose plain boiled rice, rather than any kind of fried rice.

Order dishes that contain at least one green vegetable. Try spinach with garlic, beef and broccoli or chicken with mixed vegetables. Avoid aubergine, which soaks up oil like a sponge. One aubergine-in-garlic-sauce dish can contain as as many as 1,000kcal.

Order one vegetable dish and one other dish and share them. If you're dining with a friend, this strategy will give you more vegetables and more variety. Thai food in particular includes a wonderful selection of vegetables, such as mushrooms, green and red chillies, bean sprouts and mangetout, along with fresh herbs such as lemongrass and basil.

Ask for less oil. Even a plate of stir-fried vegetables contains approximately 500kcal thanks to all the oil the restaurant uses. Ask them politely to use less, and they'll usually oblige.

Choose your Thai soup carefully. Thai restaurants offer *tom yum goong* (hot and sour soup), as well as vegetable and tofu soups made with clear broth. They're much better bets than soups such as *tom kha gai* (chicken and lemongrass soup, which is made with fatty coconut milk).

Order steamed pork dumplings rather than egg rolls – and plan to share. The dumplings are a reasonable 80kcal each (limit yourself to one or two). They're a better choice than egg rolls, which have about 200kcal and around 6g of saturated fat each. A serving may comprise four dumplings – so order one between two.

Say no to the barbecued spare ribs. With 600kcal and 14g of saturated fat for four ribs, this may be the least healthy Chinese foodstarter to go for. Choose steamed pork or vegetable dumplings instead.

Bring a big party of friends and eat your meal 'family style'. Here's a great strategy if you love Chinese or Thai food but just don't have the willpower to take home half your meal: go out with five friends and order just three or four main courses. With everyone filling up on rice (you should go easy on it), hot tea, and maybe a starter for the table, you'll have more than enough food for six people. Not only is this is a great way to sample a variety of dishes on the menu, it's easier to say no to rice if you have different meats and vegetables on the plate in front of you.

Never add soy sauce. Because your meal likely probably contains a day's worth of salt or more, resist the temptation to add the duck, hot mustard, hoisin and soy sauces the restaurant provides. Just a tablespoon of soy sauce will add an extra 1,000mg of salt to your meal – half of the recommended daily maximum. A tablespoon of hoisin sauce has 250mg of salt and hot mustard has 100mg.

Keep your main dish and rice in separate bowls. The surest path to maximum calorie intake at a Chinese restaurant is to scoop white rice onto your plate and dump your sauce-laden dish on top. The rice will soak up the sauce, which will make you want to eat every last bite of it. Instead, do as the Chinese do and keep your rice in your rice bowl, and your meat and vegetables in the bowl they came in. Using your chopsticks to first pick up a slice of meat, and then perhaps a few grains of rice from the other bowl, accomplishes two things: you leave the fatty sauce behind and you eat less rice.

Avoid coconut milk at all costs. Some of the best Thai dishes are the spicy, coconut milk-based curries, such as green and massaman curry. As delicious as they are, they contain one of the most fattening ingredients imaginable: coconut milk. From just 2 tablespoons of coconut milk, you'd get 6g of fat, 5g of which are saturated. It is safe to say that any restaurant's Thai curry or soup is bound to contain more than 2 tablespoons of coconut milk. Opt instead for jungle curry, which typically doesn't contain coconut milk, or dishes with a garlic-based sauce.

Order steamed tofu, not deep fried. Tofu is a popular ingredient in many Asian cuisines. It's an excellent protein source, packing about 2g per 25g and only 183kcal. Try it instead of chicken, beef or pork the next time you're at a Chinese or Thai restaurant. Just be sure to order it steamed or stir-fried, not deep fried, or you'll cancel out the benefits.

Don't make your starter a disaster. Do not order prawn crackers and other fried goodies. Tempting as they can be, spring rolls, sesame prawn toast and battered vegetables pack a punch when it comes to calories. Instead choose a clear soup such as hot and sour or chicken and sweetcorn.

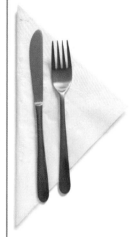

PLUS POINT
To save calories, don't let your rice soak up the fatty sauce on your plate.

Fancy a curry?

The hot and spicy flavours of Indian food certainly get the tastebuds tingling and there is nothing wrong with an occasional trip to the curryhouse. But to avoid a surfeit of fat and calories, you will need to make some careful choices. Out go rich, creamy sauces such as kormas and in come the drier dishes such as Tandoori and bhunas.

Say no to naan. You can make an instant saving of around 350kcal and 11g of fat by choosing chapattis over naan bread. Flat breads that have fillings, such as peshwari naan, are even worse, so steer clear.

Go vegetarian for a savoury adventure. Lots of Indian food is traditionally vegetarian and there are plenty of dishes to choose from. You may not have taken much notice of them before, but now is your chance to explore the menu. Vegetable dishes tend to be lower in fat and calories than the sauce-based meat dishes. Good choices include *mutter paneer* (peas with cheese) and *sag aloo* (spinach and potato curry). Be daring – try something different and you may be pleasantly surprised.

Baltis are better. Instead of creamy kormas, choose tomato-based dishes such as Rogan josh, baltis or Madras dishes. Tandoori dishes are also an excellent choice, offering plenty of flavour without the fat and calories. For example, you can save 500kcal by choosing Tandoori chicken (300kcal) instead of chicken korma (800kcal).

Avoid deep-fried starters. Onion bhajis and samosas are drenched in fat. You will be better off having poppadoms with the tasty (and low calorie) sliced onion or cucumber raita dressing served with them. A poppadom has about 65kcal, so limit yourself to 2.

Pick out the meat. Most of the calories and fat of Indian food are found in the sauces, so you can make easy savings by opting for the chunks of meat and leaving most of the sauce in the serving dish. Don't just tip the whole portion on to your plate.

Chicken and seafood are better than beef or lamb. This is a universal rule for eating out in any kind of restaurant. As long as you ensure that they are not battered or deep-fried, chicken and seafood are the obvious choice for people watching their diet because they're naturally lower in fat than beef and lamb.

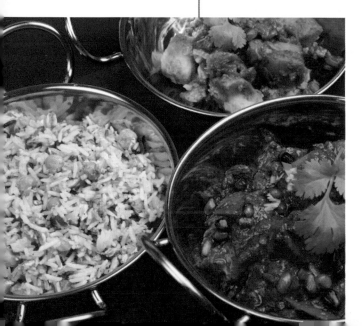

When Mexican is on the menu

Despite the deep-fried, crispy tortilla chips and the prevalence of sour cream and cheese as toppings, Mexican food can be quite healthy if you know what to order. Fresh salsa, for example, contains just 10kcal a tablespoon, and black – not refried – beans are packed with fibre.

Here's how to build a better Mexican meal so that you can enjoy the full taste experience with less fat and fewer calories.

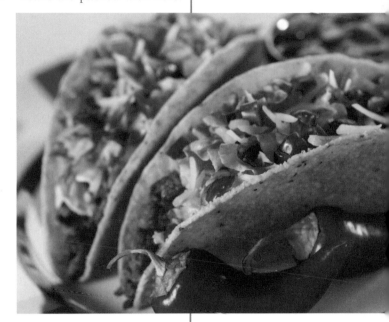

When you sit down, instruct the waiter not to bring any tortilla chips. If it's too hard to resist those crunchy, salty chips with the salsa – and who can, really? – don't even allow them on the table. A serving of 12 chips contains 139kcal, 7g of fat, and 19g of carbohydrates. Instead, order a starter of *ceviche* (fish marinated in lime juice) or a prawn cocktail.

Start your meal with a broth-based soup. Mexican starters like nachos and tostadas are so tempting, but all the oil and cheese will wreak havoc with your diet. The next time you're at your favourite Mexican spot, ask for the sopa de lima, a tasty chicken-and-tomato soup that gets a little zip from added lime juice.

Fill up on chicken fajitas. The beef and chicken in fajitas are roasted and seasoned without fat to make them tasty and light. Better yet, the fajitas come with lots of tasty peppers, onions and other vegetables. Just watch how many of the tortillas, which usually come on the side, you eat. They are high in carbohydrates, so stick to one or two. If you have filling left after that, eat it on its own.

Top your burrito with salsa and a little guacamole, rather than sour cream and cheese. Fresh salsa delivers no fat and just 10kcal per tablespoon. On the other hand, sour cream is full of saturated fat – the kind that clogs your arteries and raises your cholesterol. Go easy on the guacamole, though. It is made with avocados, which are full of monounsaturated fat. This is a healthy type of fat, but it is also quite high in calories. If you limit yourself to a couple of tablespoons of guacamole, you'll add only 4g of fat and 43kcal to your meal.

Indulging in Italian food

Making the right choices in an Italian restaurant boils down to this: watch your servings of carbohydrates from pizza and pasta, and steer clear of creamy, cheesy sauces and 'stuffings'. Italy's cuisine is healthy at heart. Big, bright salads and antipasti make it easy to include fresh vegetables, and at good Italian restaurants, fish is often on the menu.

Go for Southern Italian cuisine. Southern Italy is famous for its olive oil and fresh seafood and vegetables, and its cuisine has much less butter, cream and beef than that of its Northern neighbours. (That's not to say that they don't do pasta and pizza – they do; they're just vehicles for tomato-based sauces and vegetables.)

Don't overload on carbohydrate. Italian food is typically carbohydrate dense and it's easy to overdo it by having garlic bread with your pasta and pizza. But just take a look at the delectable meat dishes on offer. For a real treat try chicken cacciatore, or the fish special of the day. Try to have just one type of carbohydrate and fill up on a side salad and plenty of vegetables.

Keep your pasta portions in check. Pasta isn't as bad for your blood glucose as you might think – it's made from durum wheat, which is digested more slowly than, say, white bread and rice. But it's still high in carbohydrates (white pasta has about 15g of carbohydrate in just 40g), so you should limit your portions. A side serving of pasta should be just 40g, and a main dish pasta should be no more than 100g (but is often twice that).

Order spaghetti topped with tomatoes, onions, garlic and broccoli. Forget meat and cream-based sauces – make your next pasta dish works magic on your health. A study from India showed significant improvement in blood glucose levels of people who ate 50g of onions a day (less than half an average-sized onion). Other studies link garlic to increased insulin secretion and lower blood glucose, as well as increased levels of 'good' cholesterol. Finally, the US Centers for Disease Control and Prevention found that people with impaired glucose tolerance had lower levels of lycopene, a carotenoid found in tomatoes, than those without diabetes.

golden rule

Top pizza with at least two vegetables

Topping a slice of pizza with vegetables is not only an easy way to increase your vegetable intake, it's also a sensible, low-calorie, low-fat alternative to meat toppings. So go for spinach (just 100g provides around half the recommended daily intake of vitamin A), peppers, onions and sliced tomatoes. If you're making your own pizza, top it with raw chopped garlic; the sulphur compounds act as antioxidants, and the herb has a modest cholesterol-lowering effect.

Tell your waiter that you don't want extra oil. It's not uncommon for restaurant kitchens to add a little olive oil to their spaghetti or tagliatelle before they despatch them to your table – it makes the dishes look and taste better, and keeps the pasta from sticking together. But at about 120kcal and 14g of fat per table-spoon, you'll be better off without it. How can you tell if they did what you asked? If the pasta looks shinier in the restaurant than it does when you make it at home, it's coated with oil.

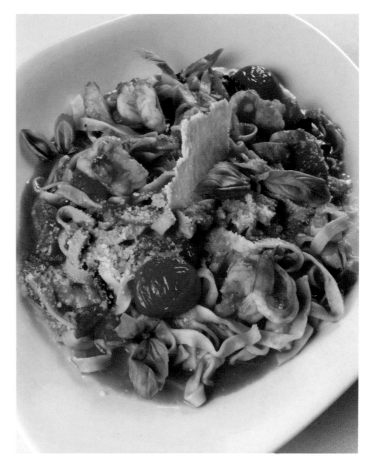

Choose red sauce over white. The type of sauce you choose is the single biggest health decision you'll make at an Italian restaurant, because it can either ensure a healthy meal or mess up the week's careful calorie and fat planning. Tomatoes, the backbone of marinara and puttanesca sauces, are a good source of vitamin C and lycopene. But if the sauce is white, as in carbonara, it means that cream is playing a major role. A plate of spaghetti with plain tomato sauce contains just 440kcal and 5g of fat (1g of which is saturated). By contrast, the same size portion of carbonara has 1,130kcal and 83g of fat, 51g of which are saturated.

Swap thick-crust pizza for thin crust. Order a slice of thin-crust pizza instead of thick-crust pizza and you'll cut your carbohydrate grams in half. You'll also save 80kcal.

Watch out for the 'pizza effect'. Because pizza contains a lot of carbohydrates and also plenty of fat, which slows the rate at which the carbohydrates are digested, it's notorious for causing a delayed rise in blood glucose. Every pizza is unique in the density of the crust, the sugar in the pizza sauce and the amount of fat it contains, so the only way to know the effect of a particular pizza is to check your blood glucose 2 hours after a meal. You may discover that pizzas from different restaurants have different effects on your blood glucose. The results will also help you to decide the portion size that suits you.

Healthy eating on the go

Fast food is often synonymous with 'fat' food, and there's little doubt that our propensity for it has influenced the obesity epidemic. A study of more than 3,000 adults found that those who said they visited fast-food restaurants more than twice a week gained about 4.5kg more weight than people who said they went less than once a week. They also had a twofold greater increase in insulin resistance. Fortunately, fast-food outlets are finally getting round to offering more healthy options. Here's some advice to help you to navigate the fast-food jungle and come out unscathed.

Read the nutrition information. Fast-food restaurants don't advertise the figures because so many of their offerings are unhealthy, but most of them do have charts or brochures available setting out their nutrition information. And seeing these numbers in black and white will show you how easy it is to trim calories and, say, order a regular hamburger at McDonald's (with 250kcal, 9g of fat and 31g of carbohydrates) rather than a Big Mac (which has 495kcal, 24g of fat and 41g of carbohydrates). You can also do this research in advance at the company's website.

Keep your favourite outlets' nutrition guides in your glove compartment. The next time you're pressed for time and have to order your lunch at a fast-food outlet, you'll have the calories, fat and salt figures at your fingertips.

Don't be tempted by the fried fish sandwich. These may sound healthier than burgers, but they're generally not. The Ocean Catch sandwich at Burger King contains 399kcal and 18g of fat (4g of them saturated). A Filet-O-Fish sandwich at McDonald's will give you 380kcal and 16g of total fat, 3g of them saturated.

Eat like a child, not a grown-up. Ordering a child-size meal rather than an adult-sized combination meal is not just cheaper, it means eating half as many calories and grams of fat. For example, a McDonald's Happy Meal with a hamburger, small French fries and a small soft drink adds up to 580kcal and 19g of fat. The adult version of the same meal – a Big Mac without cheese, a large fries and a large soft drink – contains 1,165kcal and 48g of fat.

...ued oven period for a... t half the time!	
...utrition	
Typical Composition	1 potato (approx 175g) provides
Energy	**586kJ** **138kcal**
Protein	3.7g
Carbohydrate	30.1g
of which sugars	1.1g
Fat	0.4g
of which saturates	trace
Fibre	2.3g
Sodium	trace
Vitamins/Minerals	
Thiamin (Vitamin B1)	0.37mg (26% RDA)
...ic Acid	61µg (31% R...)
...ecommended Daily Allowan...	

Order a grilled, not crispy, chicken sandwich. Chicken can easily be a healthy fast-food option – that is, if you order it grilled rather than deep-fried. This easy decision saves you 10g of carbohydrates (51g, compared to 61g in the fried chicken). The grilled chicken also has 80 fewer calories and 7 fewer grams of fat. Steer clear of the mayonnaise and save even more fat calories.

Wash down your meal with water or unsweetened iced tea instead of a fizzy drink. Fizzy or sweetened drinks such as lemonade or iced tea are full of sugar and have no nutritional value. A 230ml glass of Coke contains 27g of carbohydrates while 265ml of lemonade has 40g of carbs. If you want a fizzy soft drink, make sure it's a diet version.

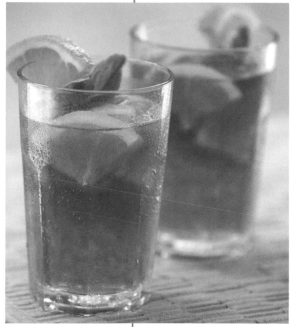

Give your bones a boost by ordering skimmed milk. Many fast-food restaurants now offer cartons of milk, and you know the calcium's good for your bones. But the milk may have other benefits as well, such as lowering your blood pressure and possibly even helping you lose weight. Also encourage family members who don't have diabetes to drink their milk. In a study of 10,000 women, those who consumed more calcium and vitamin D had a lower chance of developing metabolic syndrome, a cluster of symptoms that raise the chances of getting Type 2 diabetes and heart disease.

Steer clear of milkshakes. Some large fast-food milkshakes contain over 500kcal – nearing the 640kcal in a small hamburger, small fries and small Coke. To wash your burger down, order water, unsweetened tea or low-fat milk.

Focus on traditional mixed salads, not exotic ones. Surely you've seen TV adverts for new, 'healthy' fast-food salads. Some are Asian themed and come with crunchy noodles and Mandarin orange pieces, while others have crispy chicken and bacon pieces atop some greens. A quick glance at a restaurant chain's nutrition data shows that these salads are sometimes more fatty and calorie-laden than the sandwiches and burgers. If nutritional information is not at hand, stick to salads that are full of vegetables rather than cheese, croutons, 'crispy' meats (which means they have been fried) and noodles. Also, choose a non-creamy dressing and use it sparingly.

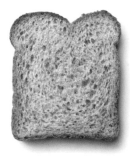

PLUS POINT

Bread, rather than bagel. Turkey breast, not bacon. Simple switches dramatically reduce the calories in your sandwich.

Making lean choices at the sandwich bar

Many people buy lunches in a sandwich shop or from the supermarket because they perceive them to be a healthy choice (and the labelling sometimes advertises this). Sandwiches can be a healthy option, if you make the right choices. However, some shops' 'BLTs' and mayonnaise-laden fillings can do more damage to your diet than you think. Here's how to make the best choices.

Before you bite into a bagel, budget those carbohydrates into your meal plan. A typical bakery bagel contains about 70g of carbohydrates – about five times as many carbs as a slice of whole-wheat bread (and more than four carb exchanges, for those who are counting). Research shows that the amount of carbohydrates, not the kind of carbohydrates, most influences the amount of glucose in the blood. Eating a whole bagel in one sitting may cause your blood glucose to rise; consider eating half of the bagel now, and half later in the day to spread out your carbohydrate intake.

Avoid the salami and bacon. You'll blow your saturated fat and salt allowance for the day. A single bacon rasher has 65kcal and 1g of salt. Compare that to a slice of smoked turkey breast, with only 28kcal and 257mg of salt.

Ask for less meat and extra fillings. A serving size of cooked meats is just two slices – a fraction of what sandwich shops usually give you. Ask them to cut the meat in half and bulk up your sandwich (and add extra flavour and crunch) with lettuce, rocket, tomatoes, hot peppers, onions and cucumber.

Go without the mayo, special sauce and cheese. Even a lean turkey breast sandwich can be full of fat if you add on cheese and fattening condiments. Simple switches can bring your sandwich back within healthy bounds: substituting mustard for mayonnaise makes it 10g of fat lighter. Avoid vague-sounding 'house' or 'special' sauces, too, which are usually mayonnaise based.

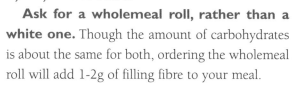

Ask for a wholemeal roll, rather than a white one. Though the amount of carbohydrates is about the same for both, ordering the wholemeal roll will add 1-2g of filling fibre to your meal.

Why not skip the roll altogether? Most sandwich shops will turn your favourite filled roll into a salad by putting the meat and vegetables onto a bed of lettuce. A large white roll can have 38g of carbohydrates – a huge saving if you skip it. Have a piece of fruit instead.

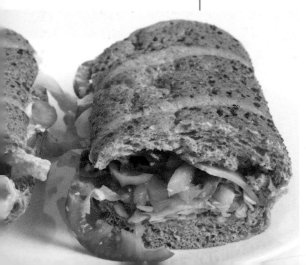

Put your drinks on a diet

Most of us would prefer to eat our calories rather than drink them. Studies have shown that even a high-calorie drink will never be as satisfying as something that you bite into. Here's how to keep your drinks from pushing an otherwise healthy meal into the high-calorie 'red zone'.

Beware of fancy water. These days, water isn't just water. Sometimes it comes in colours and has added vitamins, herbs or even caffeine. These designer waters are being marketed as a healthy alternative to regular bottled water or soft drinks. But are they worth the hefty price? Probably not. And many of these waters are not calorie free, as plain water is, so read the labels. One bottle may contain two servings, so don't forget to double the calorie count if you drink the whole thing.

Follow the 50/50 rule. If there's a particular drink you really like that's a bit high in calories, go ahead and have it – after you've diluted it with an equal amount of ordinary water. Getting plenty of fluids into your body is important for everyone and especially for people with diabetes. It improves blood flow and helps the kidneys to do their job of flushing toxins from the body. It could even lower your risk of diabetes-related kidney damage. So if you really dislike plain water and 'flavouring' it a bit with one of these drinks helps you to consume more, by all means do it.

Is coffee okay?

Every other week, it seems, a new health report comes out about coffee. Studies have suggested that the beverage protects us against certain cancers and Parkinson's disease, and it's one of the best sources of antioxidants in our diet (mainly because we drink so much of it). But there's more.

One of the compounds in coffee, called chlorogenic acid, has been shown in animal studies to lower blood glucose. Coffee's also rich in quinides, compounds that make the body more sensitive to insulin. These could be among the reasons why regular coffee drinkers seem to have a lower risk of developing diabetes. A survey of 80,000 women conducted in America showed that drinking 2 to 3 cups a day lowered the chance of developing Type 2 diabetes by about a third.

So go ahead and buy coffee from a local coffee shop – but stick to decaf, because caffeine can cause spikes in your blood glucose by raising so-called 'stress' hormones that stimulate the release of stored glucose from the liver.

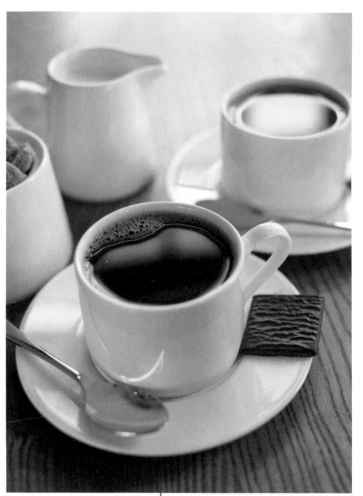

Drink unsweetened iced tea instead of fizzy drinks. You'll not only save yourself the calories, you'll also infuse your body with disease-fighting antioxidants.

Fade that coffee to black. Given the myriad flavours, fillers and toppings you can add to coffee these days, black coffee may sound rather plain – but it's practically calorie-free. A large black coffee at Starbucks has only 4kcal and 0g of carbohydrate, and a shot of espresso with a splash of semi-skimmed milk has only 8kcal and 1g of carbs. The more you add to your java, the more those numbers go up: a shot of espresso sweetened with caramel and served with whipped cream has 110kcal and 9g of fat, 6g of which are saturated.

Order your java drinks 'skinny'. In coffee-shop lingo, 'skinny' means, 'made with skimmed milk' and people who don't want to drink their calories are making the switch from 'fat' to 'skinny'. Ordering a Grande latte made with skimmed milk instead of whole milk will cut about 100kcal out of the drink.

Treat fancy, specialty coffees as you would a dessert. The more flavours and toppings you add to a specialty coffee drink, the higher its calorie count climbs – so high, in some cases, that ordering an ice cream would be healthier. An ice cream cone with one scoop of vanilla ice cream contains about 185kcal and 8g of fat (5g saturated). A white chocolate mocha with whipped cream 'Venti' contains a staggering 619kcal, 27g fat and 78g of carbohydrate. Always bear in mind that these drinks aren't refreshments – they're desserts – and should be consumed sparingly, on special occasions.

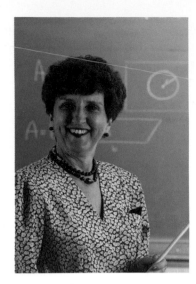

11

At work

When you set off for work each day,

you take your diabetes with you. Plan

to treat it well by eating healthily,

fitting in some exercise and

keeping stress under control

while you're doing your job.

Eating well at work

No matter what your occupation, to function properly you'll need a clear head – and that means steady blood glucose. Making a commitment to eat nourishing meals and snacks at work may involve a little extra effort, but think of it as time devoted to satisfying your most important customer: your body.

Make your lunch when you prepare dinner. If you don't have a workplace cafeteria or if the one you have doesn't offer healthy options, you're better off bringing your own lunch. This isn't as difficult or time-consuming as it sounds – just make tomorrow's lunch tonight, while you're making dinner. You'll be in the kitchen anyway. One thing you can do is make an extra serving of your dinner and set it aside for the next day. If you don't want to eat the same thing two days in a row, do something new with the main dinner ingredient. For example, slice some of the roasted chicken you have just made and tuck it into a wholemeal pitta bread with some tomato slices, or toss it with some wholemeal pasta and broccoli.

While you're in the kitchen, pack a few snacks. Why resort to vending-machine junk foods when you can bring your gourmet bites from home? Put a few items such as low-fat mozzarella cheese sticks, hummus, sliced apples, mandarin oranges, and fruit and yoghurt into plastic containers, put them in your lunchbox, and keep the lunchbox in the refrigerator. The whole exercise takes less than 5 minutes and saves you the hassle of doing it during the hectic morning rush.

Carry a cool lunch bag. If you don't have a fridge at your workplace, don't despair. Use an insulated cool bag, so that you can bring chilled meals and snacks to work. You'll can buy cool bags in department stores, gift shops and at www.amazon.co.uk.

golden rule

Eat as healthily at work as you would at home

The calories and fat you eat outside your home count just as much as those you consume under your own roof – so why are you so careful when you cook your own meals but abandon your rules when you're at work? Get into the habit of taking with you both a homemade lunch and a bit of self-control when you go to work. Tell yourself that you're going to feel great round the clock, not just when you're off duty.

Whip it together!

Your own takeaway chilli

Why settle for a cold sandwich when you can have a hot lunch from home? This one's full of protein to keep you full all day.

Chop 3 **spring onions** and crush 2 **garlic** cloves. In a large pan sauté them in 2 teaspoons of **olive oil** for 3 minutes. Add 1 tablespoon **chilli powder** and 1 teaspoon ground **cumin**. Add 450g lean **minced turkey** or **chicken**. Brown for 5 minutes over medium heat. Add 1 can (about 400g) drained and rinsed **kidney beans** and 1 can (400g) **chopped tomatoes**. Simmer for 5 minutes. Spoon into an air-tight container and refrigerate.

Reheat prior to serving.

Ask your dietitian for interesting lunch suggestions. If eating the same snacks and lunches day in and day out is becoming boring, make an appointment with a registered dietitian. These nutritional professionals have tonnes of creative ideas about healthy, time-saving snacks and meals you can bring to work, no matter what your work hours are like. They'll always take into account the foods you like most.

'Lunch-share' with three health-conscious colleagues. Lunch-sharing is like car-sharing, but for meal preparation. Band together with a few friends who are tired of the hassle of bringing their lunch every day, and allocate each person a day of the week. On their set days, lunch-share club members will prepare a healthy meal that will feed all four people in the club. It means less cooking for everyone and an enjoyable opportunity to try some new dishes you might want to use in your own menu.

Highlight healthy options on your favourite takeaway menus. It happens all the time – someone comes around with a takeaway menu and invites you to order. And of course the menu is full of choices that would blow your entire fat, calories and salt allowance for the rest of the day. No problem – that's precisely why you've done your homework and identified two or three dishes that won't sabotage your eating plan. Ask for one of those dishes and you won't even have to look temptation in the face.

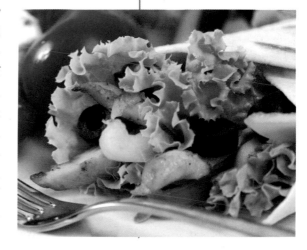

Resisting tempting treats at work

Surveys show that many people feel that they put on weight as a direct result of their work environment. It's easy to see why: we all give in to vending machines, bowls of sweets on colleagues' desks and the obligatory office birthday cake. If you're sitting behind a desk all day, the pounds seem to sneak up on you even faster. Because excess weight is a problem for so many people with diabetes, resisting the small temptations at work will go a long way towards helping you to manage your condition.

Spend your breaks in a snack-free area. The snacks that you're likely to find in the break room can make it one of the most dangerous areas at your workplace. Look for another quiet spot where you can retreat during your time off. This can be a shady area under some trees behind the building, a quiet filing room with a chair or an out-of-the-way, unused office with a pleasant view. When your usual break room is laden with cakes that your colleagues have brought in, sneak away to your special spot.

Sip cool water throughout the day. Bring two 800ml bottles of water to work each morning, and make it a goal to drink them before you go home. This is important for a few reasons: being dehydrated can cause your blood glucose to rise. Also, water is filling, so you'll feel less hungry during the day. Research shows that you can burn 50kcal extra each day if you drink 1.5 litres of cold water or more, because

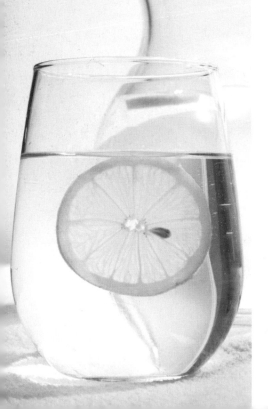

you have to expend energy to bring the water up to body temperature. Do this for a year and you'll lose about 2kg, not counting the calories you're not ingesting by drinking fizzy drinks.

Give your water a zesty fruit flavour. At the start of the working week, bring several sliced limes or lemons in a resealable plastic bag and store them in the refrigerator at work. When you refill your water bottle, squeeze some juice into the bottle, then add the slice. For variety, try dropping slices of cucumber, strawberries or sprigs of mint into your water. It will certainly encourage you to drink more.

Stock your desk or locker with a variety of teas. Sipping hot tea is an easy way to drink a lot of water and feel full while you work. Green or black teas are also two of the most potent sources of antioxidants in nature, and sipping them regularly has been shown to decrease the risk of heart disease and stroke, to which people with diabetes

make the change

The habit: Choosing baked crisps instead of fried from the vending machine.

The result: Losing about 3kg a year.

The evidence: They may seem like the same kind of snack – they're both tasty and crunchy – but baked crisps are a much better vending choice than fried. A typical 34.5g bag of fried crisps contains 183kcal and 11.3g of fat compared to a 25g bag of baked crisps which has 90kcal and 0.6g of fat. If you picked the baked crisps instead of the fried crisps every workday, after a year you'd save about 24,500kcal – the equivalent of 3kg of body weight! You'd save yourself considerable amount of artery-clogging saturated fat, as well.

are more susceptible. For the sake of your blood pressure, choose decaffeinated tea (it contains the same amount of antioxidants). Store the tea-bags inside an airtight container, in a cool, dry place (a desk drawer is ideal).

Bring your own healthy snacks. You'll have no excuse to visit the vending machine when a snack craving strikes. But don't keep too many because that could prove too tempting and encourage you to eat when there's simply no need. But it's useful to have low-fat crackers or some fresh fruit around when you're feeling peckish. And, if you have a refrigerator at work, keep some low-fat cheese sticks and low-fat yoghurt in it.

Keep sugarless mints and gum in your drawer. You can chew on one when temptation strikes. If you're due at a meeting in 10 minutes and you know there will be doughnuts or biscuits on the table, pop a couple of breath mints or a piece of chewing gum into your mouth before you go to it. The strong flavour of mint ruins the taste of anything that you eat, especially sugary baked goods. It's a bonus that your breath smells sweet while you're talking business.

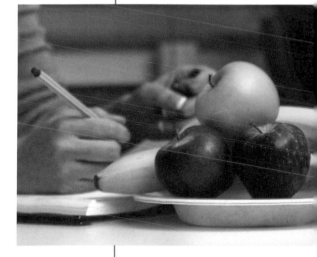

Focus on your food when you're eating. You get more work done when you focus exclusively on the job in hand; similarly, you'll get more flavour and enjoyment out of your snacks and meals if you focus all your attention on the food in front of you when you eat. Don't work or browse the internet as you eat. Sit outside under a tree, or turn off your screen and look out of the window while you eat – then you're not only enjoying your food, you're also de-stressing a bit.

whip it together!

Bagel crisps

When the afternoon munchies strike, reach for these home-made bagel crisps, which are much lower in calories and fat than store-bought ones.

Preheat the oven to 210°C. Slice one **wholemeal bagel** horizontally into 4 slices. Cut each of the slices into 6 pieces. Spread out the bagel pieces on a large baking sheet and spray them with olive oil cooking spray. In a small bowl combine 2 tablespoons grated **Parmesan cheese,** 1 tablespoon dried **basil**, 2 teaspoons dried **oregano**, 2 teaspoons **garlic powder** and **salt** and **pepper** to taste. Sprinkle the chips with the seasoning mixture. Bake for about 5–6 minutes until lightly toasted. Pack into a air-tight container.

Indulge in a non-food distraction. When your colleagues are celebrating someone's birthday with a creamy cake, the cut-up vegetable sticks that you're keeping in the office fridge aren't going to stop you from joining in. Use a bit of self-restraint and drink a cup of tea or black coffee at the celebration. Be sociable, but – to avoid temptation – don't stay too long; use the time instead to fit in something that has nothing to do with food. If permitted, spend 5 minutes surfing the internet to read about a new film you want to see, or phone a friend for a quick hello. While your colleagues are eating cakes, you'll have achieved something else – and reaffirmed your commitment to healthy lifestyle choices.

Prepare a polite reply to offerings from colleagues. Every day, or so it seems, well-meaning colleagues proffer homemade cakes or sweets they've picked up on holiday, and sometimes it's just easier to eat up rather than hurt a friend's feelings. Having a kind 'no' prepared in advance can keep those sugary treats from sending your blood glucose levels soaring. Try, 'No thanks, I've already been eating at my desk,' or, 'I appreciate the offer, but I have a delicious dinner planned for tonight, so I'm saving room for that.'

If you can't curb that snack attack, lobby the boss for healthier treats. Your office's vending machine doesn't have to be a nutritional wasteland. The company that stocks the machine may be able to supply some healthy options. Check with your manager and colleagues and then be specific about what you want: ask for particular brands of crisps and other snacks that you know are low-calorie, such as pretzels and baked, rather than fried, crisps (and you may be able to persuade your boss that snacks containing trans fat should be banished). If you think that the management would be amenable, petition the boss for a refrigerated vending machine stocked with options such as fresh fruit and yoghurt.

Brush and floss your teeth after eating. It's another good reason to get up from your desk, and you'll be doing your mouth a favour, as people with diabetes are at higher risk of gum disease.

Putting your company's resources to work for you

It's in your company's best interests to encourage you to exercise, lose weight and get regular medical check-ups. A healthy employee is happier, more productive, more energetic and takes fewer days off sick. As a result, businesses are now offering programmes to help their workers track and improve their health. Take full advantage.

Take advantage of company health screenings. Some companies host health screenings regularly and invite nurses and other health professionals to come to the office and check employees' blood pressure and cholesterol, perform skin-cancer screenings and more. If your company does this, find out when these screenings will take place and be sure to sign up. Everyone with diabetes should get a flu injection each year, and keeping tabs on your blood pressure and cholesterol are especially important if you have diabetes because of the increased risk of heart attack and stroke that comes with the disease.

Learn whether your company offers incentives to exercise. Some companies offer reduced fees at the local gym or money off sports lessons. It doesn't hurt to ask, and if your company doesn't offer these incentives yet, maybe you'll inspire them to start.

Suggest ways to make your workplace healthier. Your bosses know that happy, healthy employees are more productive employees. Why wouldn't they be interested in your suggestions for improving the workplace, particularly if they don't cost much? If the cafeteria offers too many fried foods and not enough vegetables, suggest specific improvements. Or come up with ways that the company could make healthy living in the workplace more obvious – perhaps by organising walking groups or hosting a lunchtime guest speaker. Your career may benefit, too, because you'll be seen as a team player with creative problem-solving skills.

Start a good-natured weight-loss competition. This takes nerve but if you know your colleagues are as health-conscious as you, you might just make it work. Suggest a little contest to test who can lose the most weight over a set period of time. You could set up a sweepstake with a pound to enter and the winner gets the pot. You might even organise colleagues into teams, or by department: set the accounts department up against the IT staff. Hold weekly weigh-in meetings where you and your team offer each other encouragement and weight-loss strategies. You'll be less likely to indulge in doughnuts or chocolate cake at your next morning meeting if you know that your team is counting on you to make healthy choices.

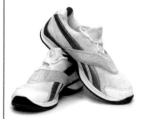

PLUS POINT
Some companies offer incentives to encourage gym membership. Find out if yours does and make sure you join.

Stay active while working

These days, it's all too common to sit at a desk for the best part of 8 hours a day – something the human body wasn't designed to do. Even if you're getting plenty of exercise in the evenings and on weekends, moving around at work is essential. It can help prevent stiff and sore joints, give your eyes a break from the computer monitor, and give you enough adrenaline to stay focused and energised throughout the day.

Pedal to work. Your daily trip to the office could be a great chance to burn calories while you escape a stressful car journey. If you don't live far away, pick one day a week or month, and pedal to the office. If you bicycle at an average speed of 12 mph – a brisk pace, but reasonable for many people – you'll burn about 410kcal an hour. Research your route, you might find an enjoyable and peaceful cycle path that you didn't know existed. Check traffic and street conditions before you leave the house, wear a helmet, and find a secure place at work to lock your bike.

Keep a pair of trainers and socks under your desk or in your locker. When an opportunity to get even a little extra exercise arises during the day – if you have to go to another department or site – you'll be ready to lace up your shoes and get moving. If you're worried about theft, keep an older pair of shoes at work.

Bowl with your colleagues. Many workplaces use sports as a team-building exercise and sponsor company tennis, five-a-side football, bowling or golf teams. These activities are great ways to burn calories; they also give you a chance to network with colleagues and managers during games and practices. Ask around your office to find out what sorts of team sports your colleagues play. Find out how competitively the team plays, and decide if your fitness level and intensity are a good match for the team. Some teams just play to have a good time, but some company teams take the game very seriously and expect everyone to play to win.

make the change

The habit: Wearing comfortable, easy-to-move-in clothes.

The result: Keeping your weight under control.

The evidence: Research has found that employees take 491 more steps during the working day when they're wearing casual clothing than when they're wearing business attire. If your company doesn't permit you to wear casual clothing every day, wear clothes that are as comfortable as your company's dress code will allow. Look for garments that feel cool while you're moving around, don't restrict your movements and wear comfortable shoes that encourage walking. On casual Fridays and other dress-down days, be sure you do extra physical activity to take advantage of the comfortable clothes. By taking just 491 extra steps each day, you can burn nearly 1kg a year.

Easy moves to do at your desk

Simple exercises to stretch and strengthen your muscles at your desk not only burn calories, they help you feel refreshed and more supple throughout the day, which will give you enough energy to exercise after work. Each morning and afternoon, do at least one of these exercises:

▶ **Leg lifts.** Keeping one foot on the ground, lift the other foot off the ground a few centimetres. Raise and lower the leg 10 to 20 times, then change legs and repeat on the other side.

▶ **Desk pulls.** If you have a chair with rollers, pull your chair close to your desk, then slowly push yourself out to arm's length. Grip the desk tightly and pull yourself slowly back to the desk until your tummy is touching it. Repeat 10 to 15 times.

▶ **Shoulder shrugs.** Many of us carry lots of tension in our shoulders due to stress. This exercise can help relieve that tension. Slowly lift your shoulders toward your ears, hold for a few seconds, and slowly lower them. Repeat 10 times.

Deliver important messages in person. Rather than sending an impersonal email or making a phone call, get up at least once an hour and talk over work issues (or bring important papers along) in person. When your message is especially sensitive or personal, or when body language really matters, the personal strategy is important. Making these trips may only get you on your feet for 5 minutes, but those minutes add up over the course of a week.

If you have an office with a door, close it and jog on the spot for 5 minutes. For more of a challenge, jog on the spot and try to kick your buttocks as you do it, alternating legs (do this for 15 seconds, then rest for 30 seconds). Star jumps work well, too. You'll burn some calories and the chances are, you'll be much more energised when you return to your work.

In traffic jams, work out in the car. First, try tensing and relaxing your leg muscles for about 10 seconds. Next, tighten and relax your buttocks for the same amount of time. Do the same with your abdominal and chest muscles. Finally, tense your arms against the resistance of the steering wheel. These simple exercises take up otherwise wasted time when you're waiting in traffic and you'll slowly get fitter.

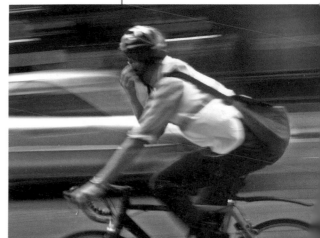

Managing work-related stress

They don't call it 'work' for nothing. Every day there are different challenges to cope with, from meeting tight deadlines to dealing with difficult people. But when you have diabetes, hassles at work can be detrimental to your health. Stress can make your blood glucose go up or down and contributes to higher blood pressure, which raises the risk of heart disease and stroke. It can also weaken your resolve to eat healthily and exercise. Use these tips to ensure that your time at work is peaceful, productive and conducive to living well with diabetes.

Time difficult tasks when you're likely to feel your best. Most of us know the time of day when we're most productive – some of us come alive at 4pm, while others are at their best in the earliest hours of the day. Whenever possible, schedule your most important work tasks during your most productive, alert times. These are the times to be making sales calls, coming up with creative ideas for a marketing campaign, or discussing new ideas with your boss. When you're grumpy or in a nonproductive slump, answer low-priority emails and do your filing or record-keeping.

Tackle procrastination by breaking large projects into smaller steps. When you're facing a huge project and don't know where to begin, make a to-do list of small milestones that need to be met, and give yourself a deadline for completing each one. Each day, choose a task that you'll complete to make sure you accomplish something toward your goal.

Take a few minutes to chat. Successful work relationships often depend on appreciating the other person, and that's much easier to do if you get to know them a little on a personal level. So build a few minutes into your morning in which you spend a little social time with colleagues. Keep it short, but don't miss this opportunity to share a laugh or story.

Cultivate one or two work friends. You know it instinctively, and science has proven it: friends make life (including work life) less stressful. Having social support at work is associated with lower blood pressure during the working day and also with smaller increases in blood pressure during times when work problems boil to a head.

golden rule

Walk every day during your lunch hour

Just 10 minutes of brisk walking could lower your blood glucose and will burn about 50kcal. Instead of chatting with colleagues after you've finished eating, slip on your trainers and invite them to join you in a walk around the building or, preferably, outside. If the weather is bad, walk up and down the office stairs. It'll also do wonders for curbing your stress levels.

Try a little aromatherapy at your desk. Studies have shown that pleasing, natural smells can relieve stress, especially when the scents are associated with positive memories. Scents that are best known for their stress-reducing qualities include lavender, ylang ylang, geranium, lemon and roman chamomile. Fill a dish on your desk with potpourri or buy a fresh bouquet of flowers and place them in a vase on your desk every Monday.

Add some greenery. Bring in some pot plants for your desk – preferably ones that survive well indoors with little attention. Studies find that plants significantly lower workplace stress and enhance productivity. Just the act of watering them can provide a brief, quiet moment of calm during your day.

Give yourself a pat on the back. When you've completed a goal, tell yourself what a good job you've done – and mean it. Praise is often in short supply at work, so when you have a chance to praise yourself, take it. You'll get a burst of energy and confidence that will help you weather whatever storms the day has in store.

Pat others on the back, too (figuratively speaking). Don't hesitate to give praise and recognition, or even a simple compliment, to colleagues when appropriate. Making someone else feel good makes you feel good, too. Someday they may return the favour.

make the change

The habit: Going for a walk instead of eating a chocolate bar.

The result: More energy and less tension.

The evidence: In a study by researchers in the USA, participants either ate a chocolate bar or walked briskly for 10 minutes. The chocolate eaters felt tenser in the next hour, while the walkers experienced higher energy levels and reduced stress.

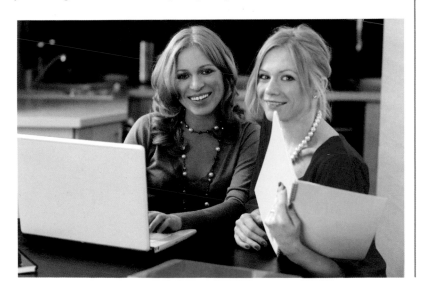

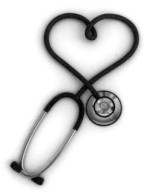

Sharing your diabetes with your colleagues

Many workers with diabetes face a tough decision: do they tell their bosses and colleagues about their medical condition or keep quiet about it? Regardless of which path you take, it's wise to give some thought about how you'll deal with delicate situations that arise at work concerning your diabetes.

Train a trusted ally to help you in an emergency. If you're at risk of hypoglycaemia, which may develop if you use insulin or glucose-lowering drugs, someone at your workplace needs to know how to help you should the situation arise. Enlist the aid of a colleague who's discreet, works nearby and is able to solve problems calmly. Discuss the noticeable symptoms you may have, such as anxiety, irritability or uncoordinated movements. Show your helper where you keep your hypoglycaemia remedies, and make sure you always keep them there. If you have been prescribed glucagon for emergencies, teach your helper how to inject it should you pass out, and keep the medication where your co-worker can find it quickly.

Prepare a polite reply for colleagues who dispense medical advice. If you tell your colleagues that you have diabetes, be prepared to be on the receiving end of well-meaning but unwanted advice. To discourage the receptionist's review of the miracle diabetes cure she saw on TV, have a polite and/or distracting response at the ready. Try, 'Thanks, what did you think of the report?' Or, 'Thanks for your concern, but my diabetes is already under control.'

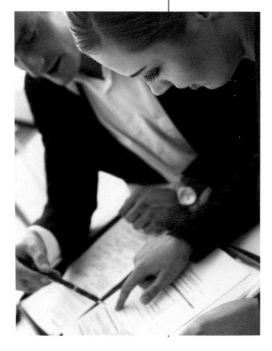

Before accepting a new job offer, imagine how you will cope in the new setting. If you have nerve damage in your feet, a job that requires you to stand all day is not going to be the most comfortable choice. Because having a bout of low blood glucose may present safety issues, think hard about whether you want to be a heavy equipment operator. Make sure that you fully understand the working hours and the job requirements before you make any career-changing decisions.

It's your choice whether or not to tell your employer you have diabetes. In general, your supervisors can only ask you about any medical issues if they believe you have a condition that's causing changes in your job performance, or if a medical condition may pose a safety risk in the workplace.

Testing and injecting at work

File this paper, ring up a customer, finish this report. You have plenty of important tasks to handle during the course of a working day, but keeping your blood glucose steady should be a high priority, too. Checking your glucose and giving yourself injections during the day can fit easily into your diary with just a little planning.

Be discreet when doing blood glucose checks and injections. You probably don't think much about checking your blood glucose or even giving yourself insulin – these are just routine activities, like tying your shoelaces. But your colleagues may be uncomfortable at seeing you draw the tiniest drop of blood or injecting yourself with a needle. You shouldn't be ashamed about doing what you have to do to keep yourself healthy, but be mindful of actions that could make your colleagues uncomfortable.

Keep your glucose checking on time by setting an alarm. When you're already working to tight deadlines and taking care of workplace emergencies that crop up, you may neglect checking your glucose. If your glucose monitor has an alarm that beeps at intervals when it's time for you to use it, make sure the alarm is set and the monitor is located where you can hear it. If your monitor doesn't have an alarm – or you don't want your colleagues to know about it – use a popup reminder on your computer screen, or wear a watch with an alarm that beeps.

Keep testing, eating and medicine timetables for every shift you work. If your shifts vary between days and nights, you already know how hard it is to adjust your sleep pattern. But you'll also have to adjust the routine that you keep to monitor your blood glucose. In a notebook, write your timings of checking your blood glucose, meals, and taking your tablets or insulin when you're working a day shift. On another page, write a timetable for the night shift. If you need help working out your needs, your practice nurse or diabetes specialist nurse can help you. Or you may find talking to other people with diabetes can give you some useful practical tips.

Carry your sharps in a protective container. Use a portable sharps container at work to hold your used lancets, syringes and insulin-pen needles. Throwing these into

golden rule

Keep a supply of 'rescue' foods ready

If you're at risk of developing dangerously low blood glucose, keep foods that can raise your blood glucose quickly nearby in an easily accessible place so you (or someone else) can find them in an emergency. These might include jelly beans or a bottle of juice. Glucose tablets are another option.

the bin poses a safety hazard to your fellow employees, and it probably discloses more information about your health condition than you may want to share. Containers specially designed for sharps are available on prescription and will fit into your handbag or briefcase. Keep the container in your desk drawer or other private area, and take the sharps home to dispose of them properly.

If you use insulin, consider an insulin pen. Disposable (pre-filled) pens may be more convenient for you than syringes if you're injecting at work or on the go. (Note that not all insulin pens are disposable; the ones that aren't require you to replace the insulin cartridge once it's empty.) Pre-filled pens are small and discreet, and you can keep the pen you're currently using at room temperature. Once you've used up the insulin in the pen, you throw the pen away. You will need to screw on a new pen needle every time you inject. Ask your health professional if the type of insulin you need comes in a pre-filled pen.

If you need a bit of support to cope with your diabetes at work, ask for it. An employer should be willing to make adjustments so that you can get your job done, as long as they're not too difficult or expensive to implement. Reasonable requests might include a place to keep food, test your blood glucose or inject insulin or a little flexibility to allow you to take a short break during the day if you come in early or stay late.

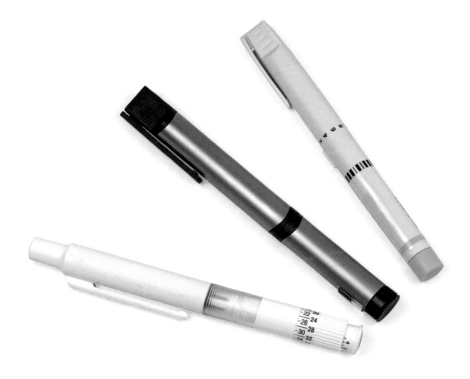

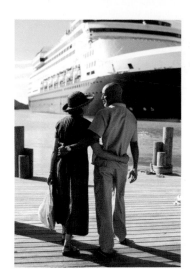

12

While travelling

We call travelling 'getting away from it all', but that doesn't mean you should take a break from healthy-living habits. Here's how to enjoy your trip, whether it's long or short, and keep well.

In the driver's seat

When it comes to quick breaks, there's nothing more liberating than just loading up the car and setting off. But you'll want to guard against some of the hazards inherent in travelling by car, from boredom to petrol-station junk food. Keep these tips in mind to arrive at your destination safe, alert and refreshed.

Fill your cup holders with nourishment. Before you leave the house for that day trip to the zoo, fill a plastic drinking cup with sliced carrots and other vegetables, or wholemeal pitta slices. Put some low-fat dip or hummus in another cup. Place these in the cup holders next to your seat – it's that easy to enjoy a diabetes-friendly snack while you're on the road.

For longer trips, buy a medium-sized cool bag and pack it with healthy snacks. Junk food is doubly tempting when you're travelling by car: you're confined in a small space without much to do, and every time you stop for petrol you keep thinking about how good a bag of salty crisps and a cold fizzy drink would be. Having the right kind of cool bag and stocking it well, can save you thousands of calories and hundreds of fat grams, not to mention money. Find one that fits easily behind the passenger seat of your car. Fill it with bottled water, carrot sticks, sliced red peppers, fruit, low-fat cheese sticks and containers of low-fat dip, yoghurt or hummus. Cover with an ice pack and put wholemeal crackers in zip-lock bags on top.

Arm yourself with sandwiches. Your cooler can save you from more than the petrol station shop – it can also protect you from those ubiquitous fast-food outlets and the crowds who flock there. Before you go, fill pitta bread with lean ham and sun-dried tomatoes plus a little spicy mustard, or make

whip it together!

Garlic roasted soya beans

Instead of chips, try these crunchy, protein-rich snacks. Most supermarkets stock green soya beans, in the frozen-foods section.

Toss 340g shelled **soya beans** with 2 teaspoons **olive oil**, ½ teaspoon **garlic powder**, ½ teaspoon **dried basil**, ¼ teaspoon **salt** and ⅛ teaspoon **black pepper**. Roast on a baking sheet at 200°C for 10 minutes or until the soya beans look dry and lightly browned.

Store in an air-tight container.

golden rule

Don't leave your diabetes rules at home

When it comes to managing your diabetes, your body doesn't care if you're on holiday or at home. The same standards for checking your blood glucose, eating healthy meals at regular intervals and getting at least 30 minutes of physical activity every day still apply. Follow them and you'll feel better because your blood glucose will stay under control.

yourself a delicious wrap with grilled chicken breast, spinach leaves and sliced red onion topped with salsa and low-fat sour cream in a wholemeal flour tortilla.

Bring along an audiobook. Reading can make long journeys pass quickly, but many bookworms in the passenger seats get travel sickness, and reading is obviously not an option for the driver. Before you leave for your trip, visit your bookshop or local library and buy or rent some audiobooks, or go online. You'll find plenty of thrillers, romances, biographies and humorous books to enrich your drive. If you're web-savvy, you can download e-books to your MP3 player. These handy devices can hold a shelf's worth of books, and you can connect the player to your car's stereo.

Keep low blood glucose from becoming a motorway hazard. Having low blood glucose while you're driving can endanger you and other motorists. If you ever feel the symptoms (such as dizziness, sweating, shakiness and confusion) while you're behind the wheel, pull over as soon as you safely can, take the keys out of the ignition and move into a passenger seat. Check your blood glucose and, if it's low, consume a glucose drink or glucose tablets. Wait 15 minutes and check your blood glucose again. Resume driving only when your blood glucose level is within the normal range.

Seek medical advice on driving safely. Diabetes-related problems can affect your driving ability, namely, blurry vision or nerve damage to your feet that makes it difficult to use the accelerator and brake pedals. If this happens, you should discuss the situation with your health professionals, who will work with you to ensure you are driving safely. If you are on tablets or insulin treatment, you will have your driving licence renewed periodically, subject to a health declaration by yourself and your doctor.

Travelling with medicine and supplies

When it comes to your diabetes medications and injection supplies, 'travelling light' is not really an option. If you rely on these items to keep your diabetes under control while you're at home, you're also going to need them while you're away.

Pack at least three days' extra supply of medication. That way you'll be covered in the event of car trouble, airport delays or an unexpectedly fabulous time that makes you want to stay a day or two longer. (If you're running out of room in your suitcase, leave an outfit at home – not your insulin.) If you're embarking on a long trip and want to bring more than a few days' supply of extra medications, ask if you can be prescribed more than usual so you'll have enough extra to bring.

Bring extra batteries. Put fresh batteries into your glucose meter and, if you use one, your insulin pump. Estimate how many batteries these gadgets will need over the course of your trip, and bring twice that number. Tape the batteries into a little bundle, put them in an air-tight bag, and pack them with your shaving kit or toiletries where they'll be easy to find.

Carry insurance against hypoglycaemia. If you have been advised to keep glucagon handy to treat emergency episodes of low blood glucose, be sure to take it on your trip. Just as important, make

A checklist for your travel partner

Managing diabetes can be a two-person job when you're away from home. Here are a few pointers that will help others to help you stay healthy while travelling.

● **Show your companion where you keep your diabetes medications.** They can remind you where you've packed them and can fetch them for you if you're unable to do so.

● **Teach your 'assistant' the signs of hypoglycaemia,** which can occur almost without warning if you do too much physical activity, don't eat enough or take too much insulin or diabetes medication. These symptoms include confusion, dizziness, sweating and shaking. Instruct your companion to quickly bring you a glucose drink, jelly babies or glucose tablets to help you get your blood glucose back up quickly.

● **Give them permission to cajole you into making healthy choices during your trip.** These might include encouraging you to walk on the beach instead of dozing on your beach towel, sharing a dessert rather than eating a whole one and reminding you to check your blood pressure sooner rather than later.

sure your travelling companion knows how to administer it. If you are coherent enough to give yourself a glucagon injection, you can probably treat the hypoglycaemia by eating or drinking carbohydrates.

On long flights, be prepared to modify your insulin use. Consult a map that's marked with time zones and count the number of zones you'll be crossing to get to your destination. If you're heading west, your day will be longer and you may need more insulin injections. If you're flying east, your day will be shorter and you may need fewer. If you have any concerns about how to adapt your injection timings during your flight, discuss the time–zone difference with your health professional before you go.

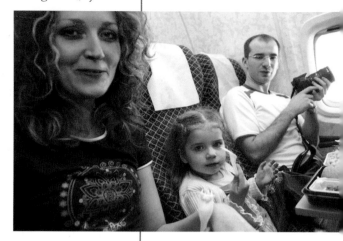

Carry your medication or equipment in its original packaging. Make sure your insulin, syringes and pens, testing equipment, insulin pump and pump supplies are packed in their orginal boxes with the manufacturers' labels. You may have trouble getting your medicine past the airport security if you don't have a properly labelled insulin bottle or the box your supplies came in. If carrying these items in their original boxes takes up too much space in your bag, pack the items outside of their boxes, flatten the boxes, and pack them flat in your hand luggage. If a security officer is curious about your supplies, this information will help to identify them.

Speak up before you get frisked. Tell the staff at the airport security gate that you're carrying diabetes supplies and have the accompanying label information to show if necessary; being ready will get you through security without incident. If you use an insulin pump, mention it, in case they want to look at that as well.

Protect yourself and others from needlestick injuries. Tuck a small travel-size 'sharps' container into your hand luggage or the glove box of your car so you can safely keep your used needles and lancets until you can dispose of them properly. Small sharps containers are available on prescription.

Guard your insulin from temperature extremes. Very hot or cold weather can affect how well the insulin works. If you're walking or biking on a hot day, for example, carry your insulin vial or cartridge in a cool bag. When travelling in the car, keep your insulin off the dashboard and out of the glove box. If you're cross-country skiing or hiking in the cold, keep the insulin in a pocket next to your body.

Useful things to bring

Smart travelling is all about keeping yourself as comfortable and safe as possible while you enjoy your trip. These items can save you from blisters and foot injuries and help you out in an emergency.

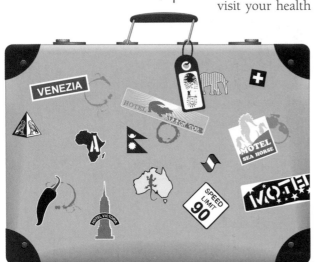
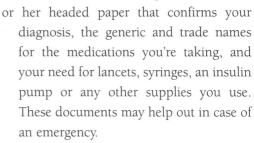

Get a note from your health professional. Before your trip, visit your health professional and ask for a signed note on his or her headed paper that confirms your diagnosis, the generic and trade names for the medications you're taking, and your need for lancets, syringes, an insulin pump or any other supplies you use. These documents may help out in case of an emergency.

Ask for extra supplies. It's useful to get extra insulin or other medications you use in case you run out or lose or break them, while you're away from home.

Pack two pairs of comfortable shoes. Wearing the same shoes all the time can cause pressure on particular areas of your feet. Changing your shoes changes the pressure points so no single part of your foot takes all the weight all the time. If you buy new shoes for your holiday that you think you will 'break in', think again. Any shoes that need to be broken in are not the right size or shape for your feet and may do you harm.

Bring shoes for the beach. These will protect your feet from hot sand, sharp pebbles and rough surfaces around the pool.

Put together a pocket-sized foot-care kit. When you're travelling, you want to see and do everything you can in a short time. But zipping from vista to landmark can not only wear out your feet, it

Build in some 'me' time when visiting family

Here's a way to reduce stress that many of us often forget when visiting distant family members: every now and again, find some alone time. Visit a shopping centre. Go for a walk. See a historical site nearby. You'll find that you're less short-tempered with your relatives – and you'll have something new to talk about to make the visit more enjoyable for everyone.

whip it together!

Crunchy lime and cayenne pumpkin seeds

These protein-rich snacks will keep for days. Their fibre is filling, and the B vitamins help your body to metabolise carbohydrates.

In a small bowl, mix together 3 tablespoons fresh **lime juice**, ½ teaspoon **cayenne pepper**, ¼ teaspoon **salt** and ⅛ teaspoon ground **black pepper**. Toast 230g of raw pumpkin seeds in a dry pan over medium heat for about 5 minutes, until lightly toasted. Pour the lime mixture over the pumpkin seeds and cook for 1 to 2 more minutes.

Transfer to an air-tight bag or container and carry it with you in your handbag or briefcase.

can make you susceptible to 'hot spots' and blisters. Although they seem innocent enough, blisters can lead to infections that can become serious for someone with diabetes. Take some padded adhesive dressings and plasters with you, along with an antiseptic wipe or cream. If you develop a blister or sore area, cover it with a dressing and try to avoid putting pressure on the area. Changing your shoes to ones that redistribute the pressure is also a good idea.

Throw in a lightweight cool bag. These bags are lined with a special material that keeps your food cool. Before you set out for the day, put a few cold bottles of water in the bag – they'll help to keep everything else in the bag cool. Then add snacks such as yoghurts, sliced apples and low-fat mozzarella cheese sticks.

Wear life-saving jewellery. No matter where your travels take you, you should always wear a medical alert bracelet or necklace to alert medical personnel to your diabetes status in the event of an emergency. One well-known company that provides alert jewellery to inform health providers about your condition is MedicAlert, which you can find online at www.medicalert.co.uk.

Step up your exercise with a pedometer. You can buy these at department stores and sports shops. Many fitness experts recommend that you walk 10,000 steps a day, roughly equal to about 5 miles, to maintain good health. Clip your pedometer to your belt or waistband at your hip in the morning, and keep yourself moving until you've hit your goal for the day.

Taking flight with confidence

In the early days of air travel, travellers looked at flying as a great adventure. Nowadays we often see it as a chore to endure before the real trip can begin. Here's how to ensure that your next flight will be safe and pleasant.

Bring your own meal or snack. Some airlines no longer offer free meals; you may be out of luck if you're with a budget airline or if you're on a relatively short flight. The meals and snacks that airlines offer or charge for are not necessarily the healthiest options, either. So pack a sandwich, pasta salad, an apple or wholemeal crackers and low-fat cheese into your hand luggage with some napkins and a plastic fork if you need one.

Book an aisle seat. You might be tempted to pity the person on the end of the row who has to get up whenever someone else wants to leave his or her seat. But that's the person who will arrive at his or her destination less cramped and more energised, so seek out that seat, and use every opportunity you can to get up out of it. Sitting in a plane seat for hours on end raises the risk of deep vein thrombosis (DVT) or

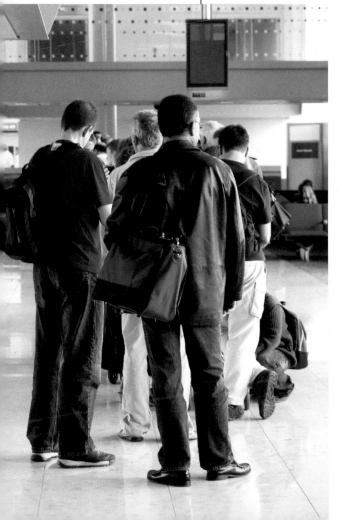

blood clots in the legs. Many factors associated with diabetes – being overweight, being 60 or older, having poor blood circulation and having a history of heart disease – are also linked to DVT, which can be life-threatening.

Set a digital reminder to get up. Time can easily get away from you while you're flying if you're sleeping or watching an in-flight movie. The next time you fly, wear a digital watch with an alarm, and set it to go off 60 or 90 minutes after takeoff. When the alarm goes off, stroll to the toilets and back, then reset your alarm to go off in another 60 or 90 minutes. You should repeat this exercise throughout the flight.

Use airport time to burn calories. Catching a plane involves a whole lot of 'hurry up and wait'. While you're waiting for your plane to board, use that spare half-hour to wander around the terminal rather than grabbing a chocolate bar from the airport shop. If you combine the calories you'll burn

Take your diabetes medication with you on the plane

Heathrow faced a major baggage handling crisis when Terminal 5 opened in 2008. Its not alone. Lost or mislaid luggage is still quite common elsewhere, as recent US research of major airlines revealed. So keep your diabetes supplies in your hand luggage. If your checked-in suitcase is lost on your next flight, it'll be the one containing holiday souvenirs, not life-saving medications. The temperature in the hold is also very low, which will freeze your insulin.

moving your feet and the calories you save not munching on chocolate, you'll end up with a grand saving of 420kcal from your daily calorie count.

Buy some bottled water once you've cleared security. The cabin crew will come round with the drinks trolley maybe once or twice, depending on the length of your flight, but you should drink more often than that to avoid dehydration, which can give you a headache and possibly raise your blood glucose. If you drink so much that you have to get up more often to use the bathroom, that's not a bad thing. Don't buy your water before you pass through security, though, or you may be required to throw it away.

Keep your feet on the move. To keep the blood flowing, do these simple foot exercises every half hour. With your heels on the floor, lift your toes up as far as possible. Hold for a few seconds, then release. Next, lift one foot slightly off the floor and draw circles in each direction with your toes. Repeat with the other foot. Finally, lift one heel as high as possible, keeping your toes on the floor. Repeat with the other foot.

For less stress, time your arrival at the airport just right. Nervous fliers can reduce their flight anxiety by leaving plenty of time to travel to the airport safely, park, check in and get through security. Not leaving enough time to do these things will certainly stress you out, which in turn will increase your blood glucose levels. For domestic flights where you're checking in a bag, arrive at the airport 90 minutes before the flight. For international flights, get there at least 3 hours before departure, especially in busy holiday times, and now you can often check in and book your seat online 24 hours in advance.

>> continued on page 216

Exercising with resistance bands

Packing fitness accessories that are lightweight, inexpensive and portable can be your greatest motivation to exercise when you're away from home – and resistance bands are about as portable as you can get. Resistance bands are stretchy plastic bands used in strength-training exercises for your upper and lower body. Stretching the latex material provides resistance similar to the effect of weight lifting. When using the bands you should feel challenged, rather than strained, by the resistance. Perform two or three sets of each of these exercises, doing 8 to 12 repetitions per set.

1 Biceps curl

Stand on the centre of the resistance band with your feet hip-distance apart. **Grasp** an end of the band in each hand. Keep your arms down at your sides, palms facing forward.

Keeping your elbows at your sides, slowly **pull** your hands up to your shoulders and return them to the starting position.

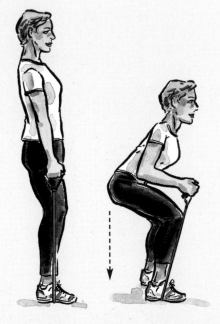

2 Squat

Stand on the centre of the resistance band with your feet hip-distance apart. Grasp an end of the band in each hand. Start with your arms down at your sides, palms facing your body.

Bend at the waist and lower your bottom into a squat, but not so far that your thighs are perpendicular to the floor. Keep your chest up, your back straight, and your toes further forward than your knees. **Push** with your legs to stand straight up, then return to the squatting position.

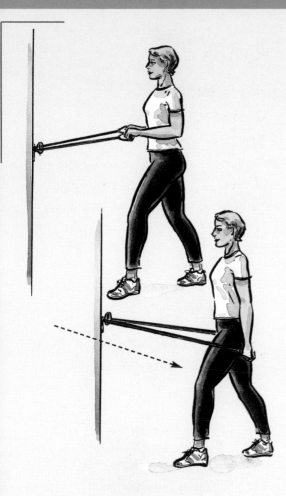

3 Arm extension

Secure the middle of the band around a fixed object (a door knob or banister, for instance). Face the centre of the band and, for stability, **stand** with one foot a little further forward than the other. Your knees should be bent slightly. **Grasp** an end of the resistance band in each hand. Hold your elbows at your sides, bent at right angles, with your hands in front of you and your palms facing down.

Slowly **push** your forearms down until your arms are straight and pointed towards the floor. Then return them to the starting position.

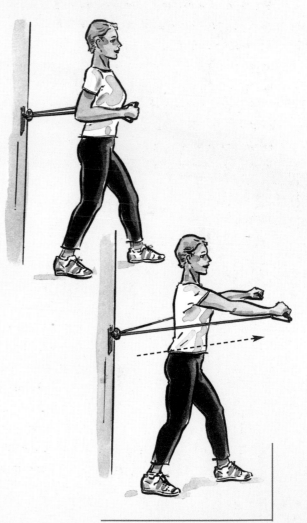

4 Chest press

Start by securing the middle of the band around a fixed object (a door knob or banister for instance). Face away from the centre of the band and, for stability, **stand** with one foot a little further forward than the other and knees slightly bent. Hold an end of the band in each hand, and let the band run under your arms. Start with your hands slightly forward of your chest, forearms parallel to the ground and just below your shoulder.

Slowly **push** out your arms until they are fully extended, keeping the hands a shoulder-width apart. Return to the starting position.

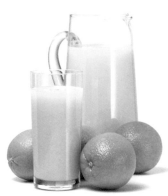

Staying healthy while abroad

Travelling to foreign countries offers many thrills: new customs, unusual foods and exotic accents. But like any adventure it also poses potential challenges. Before you depart for distant shores, take a few easy steps to ensure you have a safe, fun trip.

Get your vaccinations in good time. Book an appointment with your doctor or practice nurse six to eight weeks before your trip. Ask your health professional whether you'll need any vaccinations to get into the country you're visiting, and get them as soon as possible. Some vaccinations don't take effect for weeks.

When taking out holiday insurance, make sure you have all the medical cover you need. Know before you go what medical expenses your holiday insurance company covers while you travel internationally and what it doesn't. And make sure that your plan covers pre-existing conditions – some do at no extra cost to you.

Find a doctor abroad before you leave home. Make a list of doctors who speak your language and pack it in your hand luggage. English speakers can get a list of doctors from the International Association for Medical Assistance to Travellers (www.iamat.org). It's also helpful to bring the contact information for your government's consulate in the area you're visiting in case you need help. They may be able to assist you in finding a doctor who speaks your language.

Learn a few key terms in the native tongue. Talking to locals in their own language, even if it's just to say 'hello' or 'thanks very much', makes your interactions more fun. Buy a phrase book, and while you're studying it, make a list of phrases that might come in handy, such as, 'I have diabetes', 'My blood glucose is low' or 'I need orange juice'. Leave three lines in your notebook for each phrase that you write down: on the top line, write the phrase in English; on the second line, write it in the foreign language; on the third line, spell it out phonetically. This way, you should be able to pronounce it yourself, but if you can't make the person understand, you can just point to the translated version. Diabetes UK produces a range of comprehensive travel guides and useful phrases. Find these at www.diabetes.org.uk.

Research the local food. Other cultures' cuisines may include unfamiliar foods and dishes with strange ingredients. While you're reading about your destination, bone up on the local specialties. Seek out starters, main courses and desserts that will work well with your eating plan, and practise saying the names of these foods (or write them down on 'crib sheets') so you'll remember them.

Getting quality rest during hotel stays

Let's face it, few people sleep as well in hotel rooms as they do at home. But quality sleep is key to being fresh and alert the next day and to keeping your blood glucose on an even keel.

Book a quiet room in advance. Shouting, music and mysterious loud noises at night leave you stressed and tired the next day. Ask for a room away from the lifts, vending machine and ice machine. You'll also want plenty of floors between you and any wedding parties, student groups or other gatherings.

Bring a few comforting items from home. Packing your own pillow and your favourite pyjamas, along with other calming items – the book that you normally read before turning in or the needlework you do for winding down – will help you to feel more comfortable and sleep better in your new surroundings.

Inspect your room carefully before turning in. After you've brushed your teeth, take a quick turn about your hotel room and make sure the curtains are tightly drawn, the air conditioner or heater is set to a comfortable temperature and the door is locked. Also check the clock radio and make sure the alarm is turned off (or set for an appropriate time).

Block out the outside world. Pack earplugs and an eyemask and don them before putting your head on the pillow.

Request a wake-up call from the hotel operator. Why is it that the clock radios in hotel rooms always seem so much more complicated than the ones we have at home? Stop worrying about whether the alarm will go off at 7am or 7pm, and ask hotel reception to give you a ring when it's time to rise and shine.

golden rule

Check your feet at the end of every day

It's tempting when you get back to your hotel room after a long day on your feet to slip off your shoes, fall back on the bed and relax. Just be sure to add one step to that routine. Every time you remove your shoes while you're on holiday, check your feet for red spots, blisters, irritation, cuts or nail injuries. Treat any foot problems according to your doctor's or podiatrist's recommendations. Your feet can take a pounding when you're seeing the sights, and consequent problems can cause health complications long after your holiday is over.

Work exercise into your time away

Whether you're travelling for business or pleasure, the odds are you'll be sitting for long periods on your way to your destination, and when you get there, you'll probably eat more than you should. Plan to counteract the effects of idleness and overindulgence by getting around on some good old-fashioned foot power during your stay.

Home in on the area's best parks, zoos and gardens. Whether you're going away for an extended holiday or just a weekend, visit the local tourist information office for a local guide and scan through it for attractions to visit that involve plenty of walking or other exercise, such as nature reserves, parks, gardens and museums. You'd be amazed how many miles you can notch up spending a fun, relaxing afternoon watching the animals in the zoo.

See the sights on two wheels. Ask your travel agent about guided bicycle tours in the city you'll be visiting – or search for the words 'bicycle tours' plus the city of your choice on the internet. You're not going to find a much better way to enjoy the sights of a city than on a bike. Unlike taxi or bus tours, you can see attractions at a slower pace, and you can smell, touch and savour your surroundings. And unlike walking, you can easily see miles of attractions in a few hours without suffering from sore feet.

Take a stroll through the town square. Visiting the social hub of a town or city is the surest way to absorb the local flavour, and it's even more enjoyable when you make the stroll arm-in-arm with your partner. Together you'll be able to choose a restaurant for dinner, shop for souvenirs and meet locals who can give you insiders' advice on unmissable attractions.

Be an early bird. If your trip includes a visit to an amusement park or zoo, arrive the minute it opens. The place may be much less crowded, and you'll be able to spend your time seeing and doing what you came for rather than standing in a queue getting sore feet and a sunburn. If the place you want to visit is crowded in the mornings (phone ahead and ask if you're not sure), try late afternoon.

golden rule

Wear plenty of sunscreen

After being cooped up indoors most of the year, it's natural to seek out the sun on holiday. But sitting in the heat for too long can make your insulin work more quickly, while a bad case of sunburn can raise your blood glucose and even lead to infection. Use a sunscreen with an SPF of 30 or higher, and put it on much more liberally than you think you should – studies show most people don't use nearly enough and don't reapply often enough. If you have trouble reaching your legs and feet while applying sunscreen, ask a travel companion to do it for you, or buy the spray-on kind to make the task easier.

Hula, tango and fish like the locals do. You know the old saying, 'When in Rome, do as the Romans do'. Well, if you're in Argentina, take a tango lesson. In Hawaii, learn to hula. Wherever your travels may take you, there's an activity that will help you to learn more about the area and its people – and keep you moving.

Send yourself on a hunt for great photos. Make a wish list of at least 25 photos that you'd love to snap during your holiday. Options on your checklist might include birds or wildlife in their natural setting; a self-portrait at a cathedral or fortress; a sunrise; a landscape with no cars or roads in the picture; and a panoramic shot taken from a high vantage point. Be sure to give yourself an ambitious list that requires walking all over town to get the shots you want. Reward yourself for achieving your goal by purchasing a beautiful photo album in which to display your work.

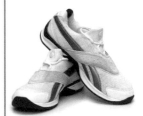

PLUS POINT
Stay out of the midday heat. Diabetes can make it harder for the body to cool itself.

Visit the museums during the midday heat. Even if you're vigilant about using sunscreen, it's wise to move inside during the hottest hours – usually between noon and 2pm – to ensure that you don't overheat or get a sunburn. Diabetes may cause your sunburn to heal more slowly or lead to infection, and it may be harder for people with diabetes to cool themselves. Use these hours to see a museum exhibit, grab a bite to eat or take a scenic trip by car.

Keep a sports bag packed with workout gear. If you travel frequently for business, stuff a small bag with all the workout gear you need, and keep it under your bed at home so it's always ready to go. Include trainers, shorts, socks, shirt, sports bra, swimsuit, pedometer, towel, soap, deodorant and a combination lock. You'll be able to squeeze in a quick jog or swim at your hotel when you arrive, or use an airport gym during a stopover. You'll also have the gear you need to freshen up afterwards.

Go to the gym or pool first thing in the morning. Business travel is filled with meetings, conferences, interviews and meals with clients. If you don't make time for exercise it won't happen. Getting it in first thing in the morning is the best time for many travellers. Your diary is least likely to be hectic then, and a vigorous morning workout can keep you going all day.

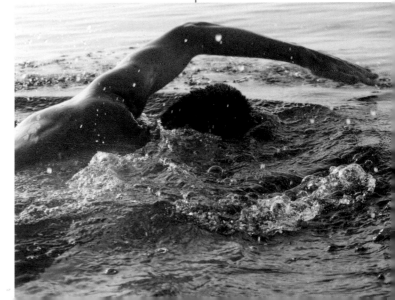

Staying healthy on the high seas

For many people a cruise is a dream come true – a floating paradise, the ultimate luxury. Apart from the pitfalls of the all-you-can-eat buffets, the truth is, cruises can be as healthy and active as you make them. So pack your trainers, swimsuit and dancing shoes, and follow these tips. You'll return from your holiday in great shape.

Aim to burn more calories than you do at home. This should be simple – you can easily fit in at least 30 minutes of walking during the average shore excursion. And on a moderate-size ship, you can log a mile with just four laps around the promenade deck, which is designed for just that (no deck chairs in the way). That's not even counting the exercise you can do in the swimming pool, in the gym or in the ocean – snorkelling anyone?

Get hold of a sample menu, or find one online. Bring it to your dietitian, who can help you to work out how to make choices that will fit into your eating plan. That way you won't be overwhelmed when you get there.

Pick out one 'prize' at the buffet table. From the outside, a cruise liner looks like a ship. Once you're on board, it looks more like a floating smorgasbord. Before you fill your plate, scan the entire buffet table and choose one small, indulgent item as a treat, so you can feel as if you've been part of the fun, without overdoing it.

Beat those germs. Its easy to pick up a stomach virus on a cruise ship. But, feeling sick ruins your day and makes it much more difficult to control your blood glucose. The solution is at your fingertips: wash your hands frequently. Do it after you touch items that other passengers touch and just before meals. For extra protection, you might want to keep a bottle of hand sanitiser in your pocket.

Sign up for active excusions. Some shore trips, such as eating at a famous local restaurant or seeing sites by bus, barely require getting up from your seat. But others, including biking excursions or snorkelling trips, provide a great workout. Some cruises even let you prebook shore excursions. Just make sure that you choose ones that are a good match for your physical abilities. If you have any doubts, talk to the activities manager.

While ashore, choose your food carefully. The food on cruise ships is usually safe, but the same isn't necessarily true when you venture ashore. Avoid raw fruits and vegetables, tap water, iced drinks and food sold by street sellers.

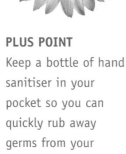

PLUS POINT

Keep a bottle of hand sanitiser in your pocket so you can quickly rub away germs from your hands.

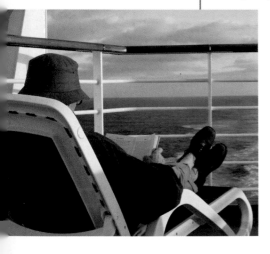

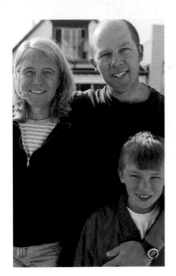

13
In your family

Your diabetes affects your family, too;

if you have to live with the disease

for the rest of your life, so do they.

Here's how to get the support you

need while keeping family life

happy and stress free.

Bring your family on board

The more your family knows about diabetes, the more they'll appreciate what you're going through as you try to manage your health and the more they'll be able to help. You should never feel as if you're in this alone.

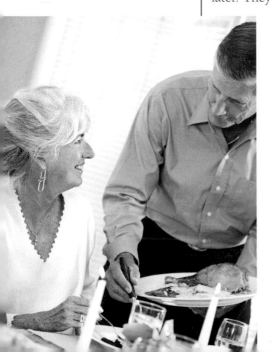

Don't hide your diabetes. Some people try to avoid informing their partners of their diagnosis, partly out of a stoic 'I can handle it alone' attitude. The truth is, managing diabetes affects so many aspects of your life that you need the cooperation and understanding of everyone under your roof.

Bring home information about living with diabetes. You may know this information because you have diabetes, but someone who doesn't might forget about some of the issues – such as the need to check blood glucose levels several times a day, to eat at regular intervals and to watch calories and carbohydrates.

Bring loved ones to your diabetes support group. Letting your partner or family members listen in and discover the sort of things that concern people with diabetes will give them a much better idea of what you're facing and the challenges you might encounter later. They may even pick up some tips that will help you.

Train your family to recognise and treat low blood glucose. Everyone should know the signs – rapid heartbeat, sweating and mental confusion – and how to take emergency measures. (Plus, the fact that people who are hypoglycaemic often claim to feel fine when they're not.) They need to know where you keep your emergency foods and how much to give you. If you have a prescription for glucagon, train your family to inject it.

Teach them about high blood glucose, too. They should know the symptoms – unusual thirst, the need to urinate frequently, blurry vision and reduced energy – and be ready to take emergency measures. Make sure they know how to test your blood glucose, and if you're on insulin, how and when to administer it.

Food and family

If you and your partner are used to sitting down to big roast dinners or Chinese take-aways, at least one of you is going to have to change your ways. Your family members need to realise from the start that you're serious about following your new eating plan. Why not get them to join you? Remember, the same habits that you're aiming for – eating well and exercising regularly – are good for just about everybody.

Eat meals together as a family. Experts say that families reap enormous emotional benefits when its members eat meals together. Family communication improves, people eat more nutritiously and the behaviour of children is better overall. All of this means that your household is less stressful and more harmonious.

Make your own healthy selections at the supermarket. If you aren't the main shopper for the family, go to the supermarket with your partner and make sure that the shopping trolley contains foods that you like but also ones that fit into your eating plan. This will increase the odds that home-cooked meals are right for you and will help you to reach your goals for weight-loss and blood glucose control. It will also reduce the risk of disagreements over your household's weekly menu-plans.

Reduce – don't banish – the junk food. Unless you do all the food shopping for the household, you may feel as if you have little control over whether tempting foods enter your house. On the other hand, you might also be reluctant to ban all junk foods and 'punish' your family. There is a middle ground: ask the family shopper to buy those tempting foods in smaller sizes – small chocolate bars, rather than large blocks, for instance, small containers of ice cream and small bags of crisps. If you end up indulging in these items, you'll at least have some automatic portion control.

Create a scrapbook of healthy recipe favourites. Ask each person in your household to scour cookbooks, food magazines and the internet for healthy recipes that look appealing. Try them out and put the best of them in your recipe file. Teach every family member how to make these meals – or at least the ones that they chose – so the

make the change

The habit: Involving your family in your healthy habits.

The result: They'll be less likely to develop diabetes.

The evidence: A major US study – the Diabetes Prevention Program – involving more than 3,000 people with prediabetes, most of whom were obese and had a family history of the disease, showed they could reduce their risk of developing full-blown diabetes by 58 per cent by modifying their lifestyles. The study participants accomplished this by switching to a healthy diet and getting 30 minutes of moderate physical activity five days a week.

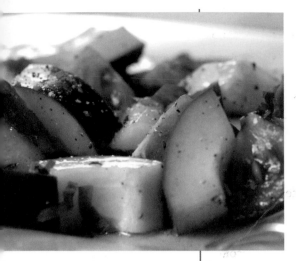

daily cooking duties don't fall on just one person. The more involved (and proud) your family members are of their cooking contributions, the more fun healthy eating will be.

Serve less-healthy dishes with bowls of vegetables. When the main dish at dinner doesn't fit into your meal plan, serve a large bowl of raw or steamed vegetables as a side dish. Take just a small portion of the main dish and extra helpings of the vegetables. Other members of your family probably won't be as meticulous about healthy eating as you are, but it doesn't matter. When you show this kind of flexibility, everyone gets a meal they enjoy.

When demands conflict, adjust your eating. For example, if your grandson is playing his big clarinet solo in a concert at noon, just when you should be having lunch, why not pack your meal in a refrigerated lunch bag? To tide you over during the performance, eat half of your sandwich on the way to the show, and eat the rest of your lunch as soon as it's over.

whip it together!

Seared white fish in zesty herb and tomato sauce

Getting finicky families to eat fish isn't easy, but this zesty dish is sure to please.

4 (100g) **white fish** fillets (sustainable types such as hoki or hake)

2 teaspoons **olive oil**

1 chopped medium **onion**

2 **garlic** cloves, crushed

2 cans (400g each) **chopped tomatoes** with Italian herbs

2 tablespoons **tomato purée**

2 tablespoons **balsamic vinegar** or **dry red wine**

2 tablespoons chopped fresh **basil**

2 teaspoons chopped fresh **oregano**

Sprinkle the fish fillets lightly with salt and pepper. Heat the olive oil in a large pan over a medium heat. Add the fish and sauté on both sides until lightly browned, about 8 to 10 minutes. Remove the fish from the pan. Add the onion and garlic. Sauté for 2 minutes. Add the chopped tomatoes and tomato purée and bring to the boil. Lower the heat and add the balsamic vinegar or red wine. Simmer over a low heat for 20 minutes. Add the basil and oregano. Simmer for 3 minutes. Serve the fish topped with the tomato sauce.

Defuse and de-stress

The fact that you have diabetes can be stressful for everyone around you. The people who love you may worry – too much, sometimes – and the time and expense of taking good care of yourself may throw a spanner in the normal family budget or schedule. Take these simple steps to keep conflict under control.

Allay family fears with education and open talk. It's not uncommon to find that a close relation of a person with diabetes is more worried about the disease than the person is. The sources of such fears are often lack of knowledge and misconceptions about diabetes. Explain carefully what diabetes is and how you manage the disease. Share pertinent books and leaflets and use age-appropriate language if you are explaining diabetes to a child. A child will become more at ease about your diabetes if you discuss it a little at a time in incidental conversations rather than in one long discussion.

Clarify your partner's role at medical appointments. Decide whether you want your partner to accompany you to medical appointments, and make sure this understanding is clear between the two of you. You may prefer to discuss your diabetes alone with your doctor. On the other hand, it often helps to have an ally with you in the consulting room to ask questions you didn't think of and to make sure that instructions are clear. When your partner understands his or her role in your medical appointments, there will be less frustration and stress between you.

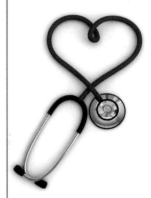

PLUS POINT

Getting your partner's backing for your health goals will ensure you get maximum support.

Work with your partner to establish health goals. Remember, your partner has a vested interest in keeping you healthy. Decide together what efforts you'll make to better manage your disease, such as a daily 30 minute walk after dinner or bringing lunch from home. When the two of you set these goals jointly, your efforts to manage your disease will be less likely to cause resentment or arguments. For instance, you might decide that you will start taking a salad to work every day for lunch. If your partner is aware of this idea, he or she might make sure that fresh salad ingredients are available and find special containers that make carrying them easier, or your partner might prepare these salads in the evenings.

Feeling nagged? Make a date with the 'Diabetes Police'. Family members who constantly offer unwanted advice or lecture you about how you should take care of your health, can drive you batty or just shut you down. Instead of ignoring the problem (especially if you are living with that person), invite them out for a casual lunch or dinner. Being in public can help keep tempers from flaring. Calmly explain how much you value them, and tell them that you appreciate their concern. Then let them know what you would find helpful, as well as what isn't helpful. Be as honest and open as possible. You may want to write down your thoughts ahead of time, so you're sure to cover all your points.

Declare an end to shouting, swearing, hurtful words and talking through clenched teeth. At a time when tempers are cool, talk to your family about the direct connection between hostility and health. Anger and stress prompt your body to release hormones that drive blood glucose levels up. If you're the grumpy one, check to see if your behaviour is due to low blood glucose levels. Maybe talking after a meal is a better idea.

Make stress-relieving 'dates' with yourself. Lower your own stress levels, and the family's will follow. It's equally important whether you're a workaholic or you're retired to find outlets for stress and for boredom, which can cause their own kinds of stress. Whether it's evening walks, sudoku, reading or going to yoga class, make the time and keep to it. You'll be better able to treat conflicts that do arise with calmness and compassion.

If you're married, put your marriage first. A growing pile of research links unhappy marriages with high blood pressure, high levels of stress hormones and depression. Help yours along by remembering to say 'thank you' to your partner at least once a day and offering to do small kindnesses without being asked. If your marriage is really in trouble, see a marriage guidance counsellor.

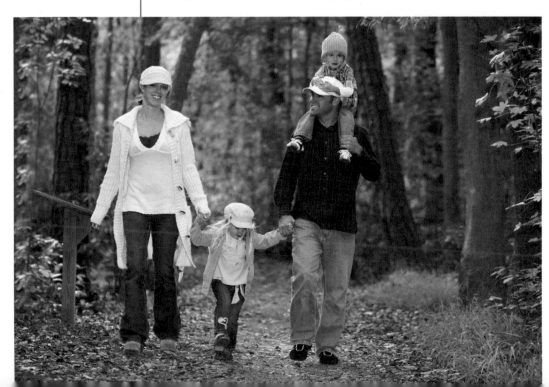

Surviving holidays and special occasions

Family celebrations are supposed to be welcome distractions from everyday cares. But for someone with diabetes, they can turn niggling concerns into bigger problems than they really are. With holidays come fatty, high-carbohydrate meals, irregular eating patterns and, sometimes, family tensions as well. Take a few of the following steps to make holiday gatherings what they should be: fun.

Stock the freezer with healthy meals. Everyone's overly busy during the holidays, and most of us want to spend our time shopping, decorating or seeing friends and family, which leaves less time to cook healthy meals. Take defensive action several weeks ahead of time by cooking meals intended specifically for the freezer. You'll be thankful later when you can pop one of the meals into the oven or microwave and turn your attention instead to writing out greetings cards with a personal message in each.

Win the food-pushing relative over to your point of view. Many of us have a pushy cousin, aunt or mother-in-law who never seems satisfied unless you have had several helpings of one of their specials. How should you defend yourself against their entreaties? If they won't accept a simple 'No, thank you', bring out the big guns. Confess that you just can't resist the delicious pie but that your doctor and nutritionist insist that you show some restraint. If you relent, take a small serving, then ask for their help – in front of others – in resisting a second helping. They will quickly come to your aid, lest they be thought of as saboteurs.

Refuse food with a smile and a compliment. When you must decline food that a relative or friend has lovingly prepared, make it clear to the cook that you are not rejecting him or her – you are just

> ### golden rule
>
> ## Keep the focus on fun, not food
>
> Most holidays are associated with certain foods (Easter demands at least some chocolate eggs and Christmas in your home would not be the same without your aunt's delicious mince pies), but that doesn't mean that food has to be the main focus. Instead, throw yourself into the other rituals that festivals bring, whether it's Halloween pumpkins and costumes, fireworks, carol-singing, tree decorating, an Easter egg hunt or writing a love note to your Valentine.

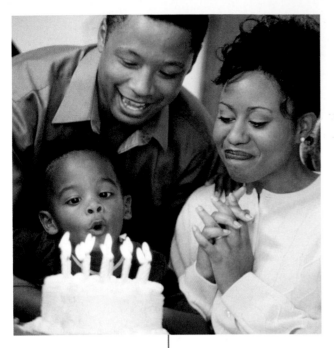

sidestepping a food that doesn't fit into your meal plan. How can you avoid hurting the feelings of whoever has cooked it? Say 'no thanks' but also add how delicious the cake looks. You might even say that you'd love to pass the recipe along to a friend who is partial to coconut cake, or ask questions about how the cake was decorated. The cook will be so flattered that he or she may not even notice that you haven't had a bite!

Modify your eating times so that they tie in with your relatives'. Do your in-laws' meal schedules conflict with yours? Here's how to compromise: say they wake up later than you do and serve a late breakfast at 10.30am. Then they miss lunch and serve Christmas 'dinner' at 3pm. To keep your blood glucose steady without overdoing it on calories, have an early-morning snack (such as a piece of whole-grain toast) before your relatives rise and shine. Their late breakfast will count as your 'real' breakfast, plus some of your lunch. Enjoy the 3pm meal and have a small snack at around 8pm. If you pack your monitoring equipment. you will be able to see how this makeshift plan is affecting your blood glucose.

Get the family on its feet. Walk about the neighbourhood singing carols, get all family members involved in decorating the house or find out where the most elaborately decorated houses in town are and trek out there (with some sugar-free cocoa in your thermos). Remember that exercise is the perfect antidote for extra special (and calorie-laden) treats.

Post neighbourhood Christmas cards on foot. After writing out your cards to local friends and neighbours, wrap up warm and set off on a winter's walk. Work out a circular route that will bring you home. Delivering the cards by hand means that you'll save money on postage, get some exercise and you may even bump into one or two recipients so you can wish them a happy Christmas in person.

Indulge in only the most special holiday treats. Leave out the sweets at Halloween, the endless mince pies at Christmas, but do save some calories in your 'budget' to sample treats that are homemade and special to your family, such as your partner's special Christmas cake. Training yourself what to indulge in and what to avoid is much like budgeting your money. Do you want to blow it on rubbish that you can buy anywhere or on a very special, one-of-a-kind souvenir? On the other hand, don't completely deprive yourself on festive days – your willpower will eventually snap, and you'll end up overeating. After all these festive holidays come round only once a year.

Choose between a pudding and extra roast potatoes. If you know your favourite pudding is coming up, make a decision: do you want to spend your meal's carbohydrate allowance there or on the main course in front of you? If it's a special day and you know you can't resist a small slice of dessert, just make sure you account for the carbohydrates and calories by cutting back elsewhere.

Bring a tray of beautifully arranged vegetables or fruit to the party. Even if you weren't asked to bring anything to your neighbour's New Year's party, don't go empty-handed. Prepare a platter that's piled high with your favourite fresh fruits and vegetables, or both, along with a low-calorie, low-fat dip. Munch on these before or during dinner, and you'll be less tempted to fill up on foods that will blow your calorie budget.

Offer to bring a dessert. Find a delicious recipe that's low in carbohydrates and calories, and present it proudly. That way, you'll know there will be one dessert at the gathering that you can safely eat.

Go easy on the gravy and sauces. You may not be able to control what's being served at a holiday meal, but you can make the turkey, roast beef and even mashed potatoes and stuffing healthier by forgoing the sauce or gravy or spooning on very little.

Make your turkey white. Turkey breast is one of the leanest meats you'll find. Just stick to the breast, not the dark meat (legs and thighs), which is higher in calories and fat. Always say no to the skin!

Add turkey or chicken to barbecue burgers. If your family hosts an annual barbecue, make less-fattening burgers by mixing minced turkey or chicken in with the beef. Few people will know the difference, but your arteries certainly will.

make the change

The habit: Staying physically active during the holidays.

The result: Gaining less weight over the years.

The evidence: A study conducted in America found adults gained, on average, more than 2.2kg (1lb) of body weight during the winter holidays – and that they were not at all likely to shed that weight the following year. (That may not sound like a lot now, but it means having to buy bigger clothes after a few indulgent years.) The good news is that the people who reported the most physical activity through the holiday season showed the least weight gain. Some even managed to lose weight.

Toast the New Year with just one glass of bubbly. You may be celebrating, but that doesn't mean that you should send your meal plan (and your judgment) on holiday. Alcohol can interfere with your blood glucose by slowing the release of glucose into the bloodstream; it also contains quite a lot of calories – 89kcal for a glass of white wine or champagne, 55kcal in a shot of vodka and 170kcal in a pint of stout beer. What's more, alcohol breaks down your inhibitions, which makes you that much less likely to resist the junk foods that you would otherwise be able to avoid. So celebrate with one glass by all means but keep some sparkling water to hand for your next drink.

Check your blood glucose more often. Despite your very best intentions, during the festive season you may be eating more, or differently, than you do the rest of the year. If you're dining at the home of friends or relatives, you may not be able to accurately estimate the amount of carbohydrate you're eating or know how the foods on the table will affect your blood glucose, so it's especially important to check your blood glucose regularly, especially after eating. Remember, general guidelines state that glucose levels should be between 4–6mmol/l before meals and up to 10mmol/l two hours after starting a meal.

whip it together!

Celebration date and walnut cake

A celebration deserves a cake and this recipe delivers one that's not too high in fat and calories – as long as you limit yourself to just one slice.

Place 200g chopped **dates** in a bowl with 30g **unsalted butter** and a teaspoon of **bicarbonate of soda**. Pour over 240ml boiling water and stir until the butter has melted. Set aside to cool.

Preheat the oven to 180°C and lightly grease an 18cm round deep cake tin and line the bottom with baking parchment.

In a large bowl, beat 140g **light muscovado sugar** with 2 **eggs**. Add the cooled date mixture, then sift in 280g **plain flour**, 2 teaspoons **baking powder**, 1½ teaspoons **mixed spice** and a pinch of **salt**. Add 115g chopped **walnuts** and stir until thoroughly mixed.

Pour the mixture into the prepared tin. Bake for about 1 hour or until the cake is risen and nicely browned and a skewer inserted in the centre comes out clean.

Turn onto a wire rack and leave to cool. The cake can be kept, wrapped in foil or stored in an air-tight container, for up to 5 days.

Makes 8 slices.

Increase physical activity as a family

Being the only member of the household who exercises is like, well, swimming upstream. But if you make physical activity part of your family's culture, everyone will benefit. If you have children in your household, remember that they follow your lead. In fact, studies show that family environment is one of the strongest predictors of child-hood obesity. If you have grandchildren who visit regularly, be sure to include them in the fun, too.

Start a new family ritual. Take an after-dinner walk to the local farm shop every Wednesday or a family bike ride on the first Sunday of the month. Soon enough it will become second nature to everyone – and something the whole family looks forward to.

Pick your own produce. Get everyone together and spend an early weekend morning gathering berries at a 'pick-your-own' farm. You'll get fresher berries along with your fresh air and exercise. And at home, you can all enjoy the 'fruits' of your labour.

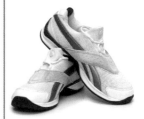

Repair or replace worn exercise gear. Nothing gets in the way of a family bike ride faster than a flat tyre or a loose chain. And garden ball games fizzle out fast when the ball's deflated. Make sure that you keep your equipment in good working order – and make sure it's not buried under piles of junk in the garage – and there will be one less barrier to keeping your family moving. And always renew your running shoes well before the soles and heels are badly worn down.

Take the family roller-skating. Has it been a while since you've been on wheels? Contact the local roller skating rink and find out its opening hours. Believe it or not, roller-skating is pretty good aerobic exercise, and it's a fun group activity that your family can participate in throughout the year. Once you feel confident enough on eight wheels, go for a spin outside – just be careful on those hills.

Map your expeditions. In your sitting room, put up a map that covers the areas in which your family typically holidays. 'Collect' mountains, lakes, rivers, trails and other geographical features by walking, climbing or boating there during family trips. Record these conquests on the map with coloured pins. On subsequent trips,

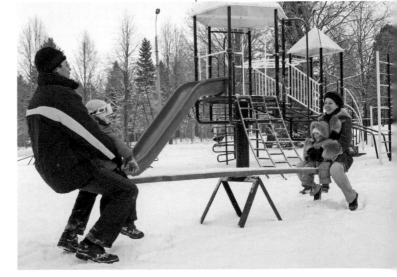

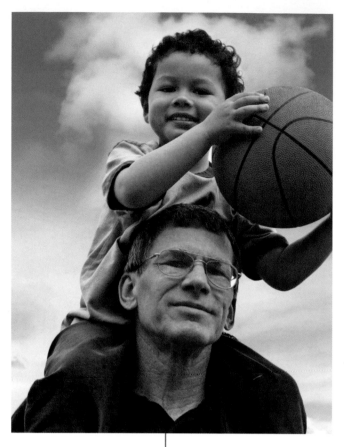

family members will want to get out of the car and experience nature first-hand so that they can add pins to the map back home.

Give your two legs to a good cause. Look through your local newspaper for announcements about fund-raising events that'll make you get off your sofa for charity – such as walk-a-thons or 5km races – and participate in such events as a family. Choose charities that mean something to yo. For example, you might honour your mother's battle with breast cancer by walking in her memory and wearing family T-shirts emblazoned with her photograph. Not only will you benefit from the exercise, but you'll also create new social connections, feel good about helping worthy causes, and tell your favourite anecdotes about your mum as you go.

Sign up for an 'Adopt-a-Street' programme. Many local councils and environmental charities run schemes where residents can 'adopt' certain sections of roads and verges. Several times a year, these groups will organise teams to pick up litter along the roadside, bag it up and deposit it at a rubbish collection site. If you need some relief in the middle of the litter collecting, take a turn as the flag person who warns oncoming cars of the road team ahead. If you live near the coast, you might want to get involved with the Marine Conservation Charity's Adopt-a-Beach scheme. See www.adoptabeach.org.uk for further details.

Encourage the grandchildren to join active programmes. If you have children in the house or grandchildren nearby, help them develop an interest in organised sports or in clubs that involve physical activity, such as the Boy or Girl Scouts. When the youngsters you're close to are active, you will inevitably become more active, too. How could you not, if you're helping your youngest practise his goal kicking, or your little Brownie needs someone to accompany her on nature walks to help her to identify plants and get her next badge?

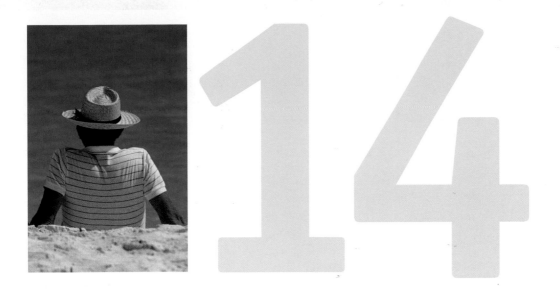

14

In your mind

Diabetes may be a physical problem,

but beating the disease is as much

about what goes on in your head

as what goes on in your body.

A positive attitude makes

all the difference.

Success starts in your head

If you were managing a business, you'd expect highs and lows, successes and setbacks. Managing diabetes is no different – except there are no holidays from it. You'll want to set goals, but expect the occasional down day and, above all, believe you can succeed at controlling your blood glucose. Having a positive outlook has even been shown to reduce stress, boost the immune system and lower the risk of heart disease. You don't have to be a born optimist to adopt a winning attitude.

Choose to fight. When people are diagnosed with a life-threatening form of cancer, some choose to fight, while others choose to give up. Being diagnosed with diabetes, even though it's hardly a death sentence, shares some similarities. If you had a close relative who suffered serious complications from diabetes, you might throw your hands up and assume you're going to suffer the same fate. Or you could take the attitude 'That isn't going to happen to me'. The choice is yours. Just remember, there is no good reason to give up. Diabetes is very manageable, and most aspects of managing it are under your direct control.

Visualise success. There are no two ways about it: taking good care of your diabetes requires some determination. Using imagery can help. Sit down and close your eyes. Visualise what you want to see yourself doing in the future. Do you want to be alive and fit and healthy enough to play with your grandchildren as they grow up? Do you want to retire and lead the sort of life in which you're not limited by health problems, so you can enjoy a game of golf, a day's fishing, foreign travel, walking holidays or whatever it is you love? Thinking about your dreams and aspirations for tomorrow can help to stoke the fire under your motivation today.

make the change

The habit: Telling yourself you can do it.

The result: Better diabetes control.

The evidence: When researchers at a US medical centre recorded the mental attitudes of 88 people with diabetes and then followed them for a year, they found that those who were confident in their ability to take care of their diabetes were more likely to follow their diet and exercise recommendations and had lower blood glucose, compared to people who lacked that confidence.

Think of yourself as a person with diabetes, not as a diabetic. According to psychologist Dr Mary Cerreto, 'If you think of yourself as a diabetic, what comes first? Being a diabetic. Instead, if you say, "I'm a person with diabetes", then diabetes is part of your life, not the whole thing.' View your diabetes as you would being short-sighted. It's a condition you have, but it doesn't define you.

Make a list of goals and update it once a month. Start with three specific, clear, short-term measures. If you have just been diagnosed, taking your medication on time and checking your blood glucose when you're supposed to, might be enough to deal with at first. Once you're used to your routine, you can add another goal, such as eating five portions of fruit and vegetables a day, or taking a 30 minute walk three days a week. Specific, realistic and limited goals will stop you from becoming overwhelmed.

Stop dwelling on 'poor me'. Almost everyone has at least one major problem to deal with in life, be it a health problem, a financial challenge or marital difficulties. If you catch yourself feeling sorry for yourself because of your diabetes, remind yourself that no one's life is perfect. Remind yourself of the future you've visualised, and tell yourself that it's up to you to make it happen by eating healthily, staying active, monitoring your blood glucose (and acting on the results).

Spend 10 minutes in the morning contemplating the day ahead. Sit with your cup of coffee, tea or juice, and set positive and conscious intentions for the day ahead and what you'll need to do to make sure it happens. Do you have your medications organised and your monitor ready to go? When will you fit in your daily walk? If you haven't packed a healthy lunch, what are your arrangements for buying one? If you have a hectic day ahead, think about specific strategies you'll use to help you stay calm, such as deep breathing. Remember that keeping your stress levels in check will help you to manage your blood glucose better. You can write down your thoughts and answers, just think about them, or – if you have faith – pray to a higher power to help you to succeed.

golden rule

Accept that you have diabetes for life

You've probably heard of the Serenity Prayer: 'God grant me the serenity to accept the things I cannot change, the courage to change the things I can, and the wisdom to know the difference.' These words about acceptance are a great reminder that some parts of our lives are not in our control, but others are. For instance, you can't change the fact that you have diabetes, but you can find the courage to alter your lifestyle in ways that will help you to control your diabetes better. When you're feeling worried, sad or irritable, remember this. Ask yourself what you need to accept and what you can change.

Get into the habit of giving thanks. Before you get out of bed in the morning, prior to eating a meal, and when you're preparing to go to bed, take a moment to appreciate the things you might take for granted, such as having a home, regular meals, clean water, clothes and friends. Don't forget to be grateful for top-rate medications and the ability to improve your health with diet and exercise. Counting your blessings will help you to cultivate a more positive attitude.

Say 'no' to your inner sceptic. When a negative thought threatens to drag you into the deep, fight back. If you find yourself thinking that you'll never lose weight or get your blood glucose under control, tell yourself 'no!' in your firmest, most commanding voice, whether you do it in your head or out loud. Sometimes this is all it takes to stop nagging, negative thoughts from snowballing into a defeatist attitude.

What's your mental outlook?

Having a can-do attitude starts with being willing to make some changes in your life to improve your health. But being diagnosed with a chronic disease like diabetes can send a person through a series of emotions similar to the stages of grief. It's not a linear process; you may find yourself skipping stages or regressing to stages you have already been through. The most productive stage, of course, is acceptance.

- **Denial:** 'This can't be happening to me!' If you are feeling disbelief or numbness about your diabetes, you might be in denial. A certain level of denial in the beginning can be positive because it protects you from over-worrying about all the possible outcomes of having a progressive disease.

- **Anger:** 'Why is this happening to me?' It's true that you didn't cause your own diabetes; your genes played a big part. So it's not unnatural to be angry about having the condition. But anger is most useful when you channel it in a positive way – like becoming determined to do absolutely everything in your power to beat the disease.

- **Bargaining:** If you're a person of faith you may catch yourself making deals with your God, such as, 'I'll be extra careful about eating sensibly and exercising if you'll keep me off insulin.' That's bargaining.

- **Depression:** 'I don't care anymore.' This is the worst stage to get stuck in because when you're depressed you're much less likely to take good care of your health. If your depression lasts more than two weeks or becomes severe, call your doctor for help.

- **Acceptance:** 'I'm ready for whatever comes.'

Now think again. Once you've successfully stalled a negative thought, it's time to put something more positive in its place. If you were thinking along the lines of, 'I'll never change', or 'I'll always be unwell', try to be more objective, specific and fair with yourself. For example, 'I'm feeling under the weather right now. Maybe my blood glucose is low. I'll check it and see if I should have a snack.'

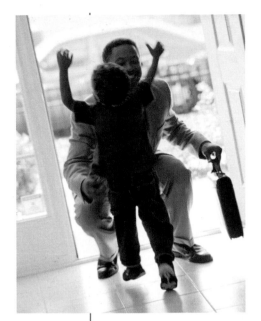

Focus on all the reasons why you'll succeed, not the reasons why you'll fail. You're eating better, you've started exercising more, your doctor recently put you on a new drug or changed the dosage, you're checking your blood glucose at useful times and, in general, you're a competent person who's succeeded at other things in life. In short, the cards are stacked in favour of you succeeding at managing your diabetes. Focus on these 'success' cards in the pack, not on any perceived 'doomed-to-fail' cards, like your weakness for chocolate cake or past problems with your weight.

Keep a positive image, a peace lily or a beautifully-shaped stone on your desk. Choose something that, for you, symbolises positive energy, tranquillity or victory, and keep it where you can see it during your day. Maybe your object is a shell from a picturesque beach or a trinket that's a sign of your faith. If you hit a difficult patch in your day, hold, touch or simply look at your object and think about what it means to you.

Put a picture of someone who inspires you on your refrigerator or bathroom mirror. People who were successes despite huge obstacles are great reminders that 'you can do it', no matter what you face. Your hero could be a legendary figure or someone in your own family. You'll get an instant morale boost when you stop to comb your hair or make a meal and you see his or her face.

Don't say anything to yourself that you wouldn't say to someone else. Many of us are so used to being hard on ourselves that we don't even notice that we're doing it. What do you say to yourself when your blood glucose rises or you forget to take a tablet? Is it helpful or belittling? If you wouldn't say it to a friend there's a good chance that you're not being fair to yourself or helpful to your cause. Think of what would be helpful and encouraging and use those words with yourself.

When diabetes gets you down

Having a 'glass-is-half-full' outlook definitely helps people to get through tough times, but sometimes a long-term challenge like having diabetes tires you out. It can leave you feeling overwhelmed, frustrated or simply unhappy. When that happens, it's time to take action. Emotional and physical health are so closely intertwined that you owe it to yourself to work out what's getting you down and how to pull yourself back up again.

Talk to your health professional. Whether it's your GP, practice nurse or diabetes specialist nurse, talk things over with someone you trust and who knows about the condition. If you're feeling overwhelmed by your medication routine or you don't understand why you're not seeing better results, don't keep it to yourself; diabetes is a big issue to tackle, and there's no reason to face it on your own.

Join an online diabetes community. Sometimes there's nothing better than talking with someone who knows what you're going through. Through online discussion boards you can find people who share the very same challenges you're facing – and listen to how they solved them. You'll have a place where you can go whenever you feel you need to soak up some support or to escape your own feelings and feel a sense of worth by helping others.

Look for a stress management class nearby. Chronic stress might be especially harmful to people with diabetes because it can raise blood glucose and shelve your motivation to eat healthily and exercise. Moreover, depression, which is a common response to stress, raises the risk of heart disease. When researchers provided more than 100 people with diabetes education sessions – some with and some without stress-relief training – the blood glucose of those who got the stress-relief training improved significantly compared to that of the others. The NHS runs the Expert Patient Programme (EPP), which is specially for people living with chronic conditions and the curriculum includes problem solving, coping with stress and relaxation techniques. Found out more at www.epp.nhs.uk.

make the change

The habit: Exercising whether you feel like it or not.

The benefit: A significantly improved mood.

The evidence: Numerous studies make it clear that exercise helps to lift depression if you do it regularly. In a study of more than 150 men and women aged 50 and over with major depression, regular aerobic exercise over the course of four months (30 minutes of moderately intense walking or jogging three times a week) was shown to be just as effective as antidepressant medications. A single exercise session can also boost your mood and help to give you the energy to do it again.

Angry? Scared? Pretend that you are a caring friend, and write yourself a letter. You will have days when you just don't want to have diabetes. That's completely normal. It's when you bury your worries, fears and frustrations without addressing them that they eventually get bigger. It's great to be able to call a friend when you're feeling low, but if no one is around, be your own best friend. Find a piece of paper, or sit down at your email, and send yourself a message. What would you say to someone who was feeling a bit down just like you are? Be kind, gentle and supportive.

Lift your chest and roll your shoulders back and down for an instant boost. An uplifted posture can actually lead to an uplifted attitude. Slumping reinforces a defeated state of mind.

Wear bright colours to improve your mood. It sounds trite, but it can really work. If you're used to wearing beige, grey or black, find a shirt that's red or lime green – and wear it with a smile. Other people will perceive a more positive attitude in you, and their perceptions can actually 'colour' your real mood a little brighter.

Write down five things you like about yourself. Keep adding to your list regularly, whenever you think of a strength or positive quality. Include things you are good at doing, such as knitting, cooking or being funny. If you get a new compliment, add it. On days when you feel as if your diabetes is getting the better of you, pull out your list – reviewing it will remind you that you are not your disease, and that having diabetes doesn't mean you're a failure.

Ask your partner or a close friend what they love about you. Sometimes when you're feeling really down it can be hard to think of anything nice to say about yourself. That's when talking to someone you trust can really help. Consider writing down what your partner or friend tells you, or ask them to send it an email or letter that you can read whenever you need a boost.

Back out of one activity. If you're having a rough day and feeling overwhelmed, go easy on yourself. If you have a mental to-do list, prioritise the items and move the bottom one to a day or two later. If your mother rings, tell her honestly that you don't have time to talk and will call her back tomorrow when you can spend more time with her on the phone.

Put your legs up on a wall to lower stress. Legs-up-the-wall is a favourite of yoga practitioners. They say that this pose not only relieves tired, cramped feet and legs, it also relieves stress. Place a pillow next to a wall and position yourself so your hips and lower back are on the pillow, your head and shoulders are on the floor, and

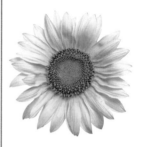

PLUS POINT
Reminding yourself that you are not your disease, and that having diabetes doesn't mean you're a failure, will help you to stay more positive.

your legs are resting against the wall. Your body will be in the shape of an L. Close your eyes and breathe deeply for about a minute. If having your legs straight up a wall is uncomfortable, you can do the move by draping your legs over the back or side of a sofa or chair.

Write down your exact fears. Are you feeling scared that something terrible might happen as a consequence of your diabetes? Don't let a vague sense of anxiety eat away at you. Work out exactly what it is you're afraid of and write it down. Then ask yourself how likely this scenario really is and what steps you can take to prevent it. Your health professional can help you to put your finger on both.

The diabetes-depression link

Having diabetes doesn't just try your emotional resources, it actually makes you more prone to depression. Scientists aren't sure why, but 20 per cent of people with diabetes experience it. The link may be insulin resistance, which can raise the level of the stress hormone cortisol in the body – and high cortisol levels have been associated with depression. The happy news: getting treatment for either depression or diabetes will help the other condition, too.

While everyone has the occasional bad day when they feel so wiped out that they don't have the energy to make a healthy salad for lunch or go out for a walk, you should be aware of when your symptoms mean something more serious. If you've been experiencing five or more of the following signs and symptoms for two weeks or longer, you could be clinically depressed and should see a doctor or qualified mental health professional for assessment and help.

- You feel persistently sad or anxious.

- Your sleep patterns have changed (wanting to sleep all the time or not being able to fall or stay asleep).

- You're experiencing a loss of appetite and weight loss, or an increase in appetite and weight gain.

- You no longer like or take an interest in activities you used to enjoy.

- You are frequently restless or irritable.

- You have difficulty concentrating, remembering or making decisions.

- You feel constantly tired or drained of energy.

- You constantly feel guilty, hopeless or worthless.

- You are thinking about suicide or death.

Can't figure out what's eating you? HALT! It's an oldie but good-ie: whenever something's eating at you – you're irritable, feeling sad or can't shake a feeling of doom – stop and ask yourself if you are Hungry, Angry, Lonely or Tired (HALT). If it's been too long since your last meal, you might be feeling irritable because your blood glucose is low. If it's anger you're feeling, you need to pinpoint what it is that has upset you. Lonely? Phone a friend. Finally, have you been getting enough sleep? Being over-tired can throw off your mood.

Buy lemon or orange-scented potpourri. The aroma of citrus has been found in studies to boost mood and reduce anxiety. You can find aromatherapy oils in health food stores, or look for citrus-scented potpourri, candles or incense sticks in gift shops. Keep several small bowls around your house.

Plant a herb garden. Rosemary and peppermint are two plants that have been shown to perk you up, with the added bonus of suppressing the appetite. Lavender is known to have a calming effect. Plant these herbs in large pots in your garden and take cuttings to keep in a small glass of water in your kitchen. You'll enjoy their scent every time you go near your fridge.

Slowly blow out an imaginary candle when you feel stressed. Deep breathing elicits a relaxation response in your body. Unfortunately, most of us take short, shallow breaths – especially when we're feeling anxious – that add to our stress levels by robbing the body of needed oxygen. Counteract this tendency by pretending that there's a candle about a metre in front of you. Take a slow deep breath in, then exhale slowly to blow it out. Repeat three to five times.

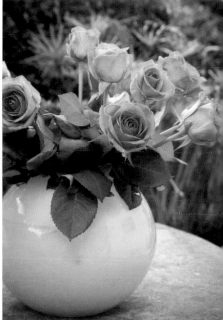

Look at something green at least once a day. Nature's a proven stress reliever and mood booster, and there's no need to go further than your own garden to get the benefits. Pick up and examine a pretty leaf or flower, or watch the birds. Taking a time out to contemplate nature gives your mind a chance to relax and refresh.

Have weekly laugh-ins. Getting together with a rowdy group of friends, making a date with your partner to go see a comedian, or just taking yourself out to a comedy or renting a funny DVD can perk you up when you are feeling down. Laughing boosts your heart health, according to an American study. Researchers found that of 300 adults, those who had heart disease were 40 per cent less likely to laugh than those without heart troubles.

Blow your top? Remember that you are human and humans make mistakes. It's okay – tomorrow is another day.

Overcoming obstacles

Have you ever watched a hurdler on the track? Those sportsmen and women propel their bodies over hurdles as if they weren't even there. Sooner or later, you're bound to run into your own hurdles when trying to take good care of your diabetes. They come with the territory. The trick is to set yourself up to fly over them so you don't end up face-down on the track.

Get enough sleep. Anyone who's sleep-deprived will cope badly with challenges. If you're well rested, you'll be more resilient and better able to face the issues that come your way with a confident 'I can handle this' attitude.

Attend diabetes education sessions. Most local diabetes services hold regular diabetes education programmes (often called 'structured education') to which you should be invited, especially if you're newly diagnosed with diabetes. These sessions cover all the

---

Getting to the bottom of diabetes burnout

Many people newly diagnosed with diabetes start out motivated to make all the necessary changes to take care of themselves. But as time goes by, it's common to start feeling drained or overwhelmed, something experts refer to as 'diabetes burnout'. Determining your level of burnout is key to relighting your fire, says Dr William Polonsky, diabetes psychologist and author of *Diabetes Burnout*.

How burnt-out are you?

Ask yourself if the six statements below are true or false.

● **1.** My diabetes is taking up too much of my mental and physical energy every day.

● **2.** I feel too exhausted or 'burnt-out' by the constant effort that it takes to manage my diabetes.

● **3.** I feel as if I am often failing with my diabetes regimen.

● **4.** I feel as if diabetes controls my life.

● **5.** I'm not motivated to keep up with my diabetes treatment plan.

● **6.** I feel completely overwhelmed about my diabetes.

If you answered true to more than two of the above, you may be experiencing burnout. Your first step is to talk to a health professional in whom you feel you can confide. Maybe your medications or injections can be adjusted so that you don't have to have so many throughout your day. Or maybe counselling will help you to learn new strategies for easing stress and improving your mood.

aspects of diabetes and give you plenty of time to ask questions and learn from other people in the same situation as you.

Join a diabetes support group. Remember, you are far from alone in this battle. There are 180 million people worldwide who have diabetes. Take advantage of it. Studies show that people who have support are more resistant to the damage of stress than those who go it alone. Ask your doctor, check at your local hospital or search online at www.diabetes.org.uk for a local support group. You'll find plenty of people who've faced similar obstacles and found solutions.

Work with your doctor. Don't be afraid to talk through your problems with your doctor. Do you feel that your diabetes medication is causing you to gain weight? Weight gain is indeed a side effect of some diabetes drugs. Your doctor might be able to switch you to another.

Role-play difficult situations. If you dread being asked about why you won't eat cake or drink alcohol, if you feel as if you can't ask the doctor the questions you want answered, or you have an overbearing family member whom you don't know how to confront, practise handling the situation next time with a close friend or with a counsellor playing the other part. This way you can fine-tune your approach before you have to use it.

Empower yourself with information. Ignorance is not always bliss, especially for people with diabetes. When your blood glucose fluctuates wildly, or you get dizzy for no apparent reason, it can be scary. Ask your health professional what could be causing the problem and what you can do about it. Remember that knowledge is power.

Too many doughnuts in your day? Work with a dietitian. Sticking to a healthy eating plan can be a major bugbear for many people. If you are struggling with food, ask for a referral to a dietitian. This expert will analyse how you are eating, help you to pinpoint your pitfalls and offer suggestions for healthier meals and strategies for overcoming temptations.

golden rule

Confront your fears about insulin before you need it

More than half the people with Type 2 diabetes will eventually need insulin. This is more likely the longer you live with diabetes. Discussing this with your health professional before it happens can help allay your fears. The fact is, it isn't really the insulin or the needles that scare most people; it's what they stand for – a worsening of this progressive disease. If your health professional does suggest insulin, it's probably because your blood glucose is too high. Insulin helps you to regain control and can improve your health and the way you feel, immensely. Keeping your blood glucose under better control will slash your risk of serious diabetes-related complications. Discuss your fears at your next appointment.

Stay motivated

Having diabetes requires daily attention: checking your blood glucose, taking your medications, watching your diet, getting exercise. All of this requires motivation. The real challenge is maintaining that enthusiasm to take good care of yourself in the long term. Use these inspirational strategies and incentives to keep you going.

Give yourself a gold star whenever you achieve even the smallest success. If you made it out of the door for a walk (even if it was just 10 minutes), if you lost half a kilo or your blood glucose results were a little steadier this week, give yourself recognition. Buy a sheet of gold star stickers from an office supply shop and put them in your blood glucose log, your food log or your exercise log – wherever one belongs. Success breeds more success, especially when you feel like you're on a roll.

Don't cancel that clinic appointment. Staying on top of your medical care will lower your risk of complications, injuries and illness. This includes regular check-ups at the dentist's and optician's.

If you're trying to lose weight, keep a food diary. People with diabetes who are trying to shed extra pounds are more successful if they keep a written record of their daily food intake.

Get in touch with supportive friends once a week. Having supportive friends with whom you can share small successes, such as avoiding chips for a week or going walking for 10 minutes on a busy day, can help you feel empowered and capable. Create a group of email contacts, or have one or two friends you can phone at least once a week.

Keep a daily journal. You don't have to write page after page of deep and meaningful musings. But it is worth writing something down every day to keep you centred and focused on your goals. Include how you felt for most of the day and note any highs or lows. If you write regularly, then you'll also have somewhere to write more profound and personal thoughts when they occur to you.

Develop your own mantra. Repeat it to yourself any time you're feeling grumpy, stressed or low. The phrase can be as simple

Signs of success

When you have diabetes, signs that you're managing it well go beyond your blood glucose results. Include any of these in your mental 'success log'.

- Lower blood glucose peaks
- Fewer episodes of hypoglycaemia
- Improved cholesterol levels
- Lower blood pressure
- More energy
- Better-fitting clothes
- A smaller waist
- Improved moods
- Better sleep
- Greater stamina
- Higher self-esteem

golden rule

Remember what's at stake

The way to avoid debilitating complications of diabetes is to keep your blood glucose levels steady by taking your medicines or insulin and by following the lifestyle tips in this book. The good news: it works. The UK Prospective Diabetes Study, a ten year study of over 5,000 people with newly diagnosed Type 2 diabetes, found that eye damage, kidney damage and nerve damage were reduced significantly in study participants who kept their blood glucose under tight control (a median HbA1c of 7 per cent). The study also found that aggressive control of high blood pressure effectively reduced cardiovascular complications and retinopathy in people with Type 2 diabetes.

as 'Don't worry about little things'. If you can't think of anything, search for inspirational quotes on the internet. If you're anxious, maybe the Swedish proverb: 'Worry often gives a small thing a big shadow' will help. If you're feeling blue, maybe the Confucius saying, 'Our greatest glory is not in never falling, but in rising every time we fall', will speak to you. And there's no one better at pure inspiration and example than Ghandi, who said, 'My life is my message'.

Do a crossword, sudoku or jigsaw puzzle. When your efforts to bring down your blood glucose or lose weight just aren't showing results (yet), it can really leave you feeling frustrated. Sometimes the best thing to do is to forget all about your diabetes for a short time and distract yourself with a crossword puzzle or other game or activity that has a finishing point. You'll get a break from what's bothering you and have a reminder that there are some things within your control.

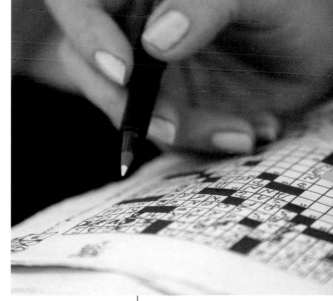

Watch a comedy or nature programme, not a tearjerker. If you've been having trouble with dishes of sweets at work or too much pasta on spaghetti night, avoid the weepie at the cinema. An Australian study found that women who

whip it together!

Double-rich chocolate pudding treat

When you want a little reward for a week's worth of healthy eating, look to this rich, creamy treat. Remember, nutritionists say it's good to enjoy your favourite foods once in a while, in moderation, so you don't end up feeling deprived.

In a heavy saucepan, combine 60g **Splenda**, 3 tablespoons **flour** and 3 tablespoons **cocoa powder**. Stir in 530ml **skimmed milk** and cook over medium heat until thickened and bubbly. Cook and stir for 1 minute. Remove from the heat. Stir in 25g grated **dark chocolate**, 2 teaspoons **butter**, and 1½ teaspoons **vanilla extract**. Spoon into dishes, cover with cling film and chill.

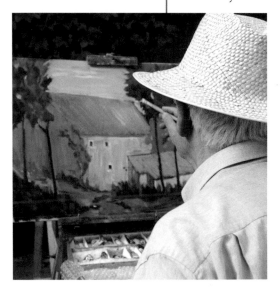

watched a sad documentary were much more likely to overindulge on chocolates than a group that watched a travel film. Another study from the University of Mississippi found that people munched nearly 30 per cent more buttered popcorn when they watched *Love Story* compared to when they saw the comedy *Sweet Home Alabama*.

Timetable 15 minutes every day to do absolutely nothing. Write it in your planner or set up a repeating break on your computer calendar. Whether you use the time to just sit quietly, to take an easy stroll or to repeat a positive phrase to yourself, having a few minutes time off refreshes your mind and helps you to let go of stress or niggling worries. Taking small breaks from your tasks can even give you more energy to tackle them.

Join an evening class for pure fun. Be it yoga, painting, pottery, cooking or belly-dancing, it can help you avoid feeling as if your whole life is about your diabetes. You'll also tap into your creative side, which is always a surefire way to feel more energised and upbeat.

Connect with a place of worship every weekend. Staying close to your faith on a regular basis can help you socially and emotionally. You'll have the opportunity to connect to others who share your beliefs, as well as time to be contemplative about your purpose in life. If religion isn't for you, a meditation or other support group might offer the same sort of community.

Do a good deed at least once a day. Take the time to hold a door open for someone who's carrying loads of bags, bring flowers to a neighbour who is housebound or simply pay someone a compliment. Doing something nice for someone else is a great way to perk yourself up when you are feeling low. And it's certain to give the recipient a lift, too.

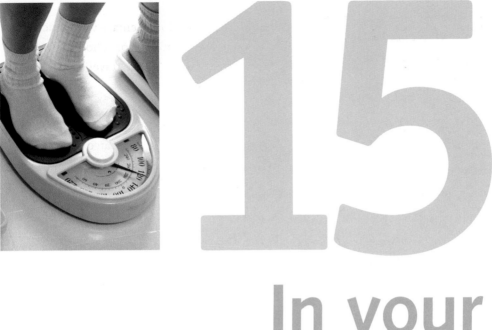

15

In your life

Everyone becomes unwell now and

then, and has problems to tackle,

such as weight gain or smoking.

It's all part of life's ups and downs.

Read on to discover ways to keep

your life on a healthy track.

Find your focus

You make time for your clinic appointments and check your blood glucose levels regularly. Hopefully you also make time to cook and eat healthy meals and to fit in some exercise several days a week. But you need 'you time' on a regular basis, too – time for relaxation and quiet contemplation. You should also nurture your soul to keep stress and depression – two significant enemies of people with diabetes – at bay.

Go 'on strike' from your life for a week. Do you have too much on your to-do list, and not enough time in which to do it? Let everything go – the errands, laundry, housework and whatever else is causing you stress – for the next seven days. When you find that life goes on even if you don't pick up your dry cleaning or dust your vertical blinds, you'll have a new perspective on whether it's worth driving yourself mad trying to get it all done. Failing to do some chores, such as supermarket shopping, can create problems. But letting a few things go will relax you and help you to work out the priorities in your life.

Carve your exercise in stone. When life starts to burst at the seams, it may be tempting to let your exercise plans slide. But on no account do so; abandon something else instead. In the end, exercise actually boosts your energy levels. It also helps to melt away stress. In one published study, getting aerobic exercise for 35 minutes three times a week had the same beneficial effects on stress and depression as attending stress management sessions for 90 minutes each week. Exercise is also an excellent way to vent your frustrations.

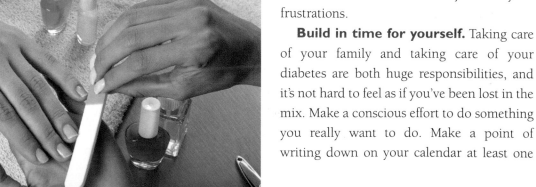

Build in time for yourself. Taking care of your family and taking care of your diabetes are both huge responsibilities, and it's not hard to feel as if you've been lost in the mix. Make a conscious effort to do something you really want to do. Make a point of writing down on your calendar at least one self-indulgent diversion every week. Treat these as the important appointments that they are, and make sure that you keep them. You might plan lunch with a close friend, a car show, a film by yourself or a whole Saturday morning working in your garden.

Take up a hobby in which you get moving and meet people. Few things are more energising than meeting new friends. But it may take a bold move on your part to get out there and do it. If, for instance, you have always wanted to try rock climbing, go for it, even if you think you may be one of the older participants. You never know who you might meet at the climbing wall (and keep in mind that it's good to have a few friends who are younger than you) and their encouragement could be priceless. Alternatively, make model airplanes and fly them at a local club, take up horse riding or join a group that re-enacts historic battles – you'll probably make friends from all walks of life, and fuel a passion that will put some zest back into your life.

If you're feeling overwhelmed, see a counsellor. Some of the happiest, most successful people you can name have used a therapist, counsellor or psychologist to get them through stressful times. Ask your health professionals about finding a counsellor who has experience in dealing with issues related to diabetes – they get enquiries like that all of the time. You could also contact emotional support helplines, such as the Samaritans, or talk to your priest.

Become a regular at your house of worship. Researchers say that practising your faith regularly can pay off not just emotionally but also physically. One survey found that people who did not attend a place of worship every week had a 21 per cent greater chance of dying from circulatory diseases (to which diabetes makes you particularly vulnerable) than people who did. A study of stroke survivors revealed that the more religious the person was, the less likely he or she was to have anxiety or depression, both of which can hinder recuperation. Researchers suspect that people who attend a place of worship regularly benefit from a stronger social network and receive more support than people who don't.

golden rule

Try to divert your friends away from restaurants

If you and your friends are stuck in the rut of meeting for meals out, it's time to shake things up. Seek out opportunities to spend time together that have more to do with fun and activity than with food. Decide as a group to join a bowling league or learn to play tennis, or get together at someone's house to discuss books. Become the 'what's happening' expert of your group by scouring the entertainment listings of your newspaper, checking community websites, and keeping up with the calendars at local health clubs and community centres.

The power of prayer

Want to live seven years longer? Start praying. This is no joke; seven years is the increase in lifespan you can expect if you nurture your soul and your health through prayer, faith and religious involvement, according to various studies. For one thing, research shows a strong connection between heart health and religious faith. In one study, people who went into open-heart surgery and reported feeling strength and comfort from their religion were three times more likely to survive the surgery than people with no such spiritual grounding. If there's a placebo effect at work here – if people get better because they believe they will – who's to argue with the benefits? Whether praying calms you, gives you hope or helps you to look after your inner self, if you feel you're getting something out of it, it's time well spent.

Keep your closest pals on speed dial. It sounds odd to say that having close friends is an important factor in controlling your diabetes, but it's true in several ways. Having people around you who care about you could make the difference between sticking to your disease management efforts and letting them slide. Friends who care about you are encouraging workout partners and will keep in mind your dietary needs when they invite you to their dinner party. When you have a strong emotional support system, you have a greater sense of identity – within a community and as an individual – which helps you weather whatever emotional difficulties life throws your way.

Lend a hand to those who need one. There are hundreds of people in your community who need you, and helping them could help you in ways you'd never imagine. The most important thing you'll glean from volunteering is perspective – that having diabetes, on the grand scale of things, is not as big a burden to bear as what some others have to endure. Volunteering at a soup kitchen or coaching a football team at a local youth club will not only lend perspective, it may get you moving around more.

Adopt a pet. Pet ownership is known to lower blood pressure, reduce stress and make people feel less lonely. Exactly how people benefit from their relationships with pets is not fully understood, but scientists suspect that this bond fulfils a human need to be close to other living beings. In a German survey of 10,000 people, those who owned pets required 10 per cent fewer doctor's appointments over a five-year period than people who didn't. A survey in the USA showed that heart attack victims were twice as likely to survive for a year when they looked after a pet at home.

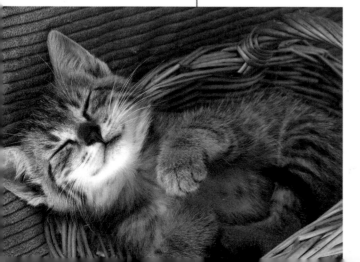

Prepare for sick days

You wake up with a temperature, a stuffy nose or a sore throat. Your first instinct may be to phone in sick to work or to cancel other plans you had for the day. Your second instinct should be to take care of yourself and your diabetes, since being unwell can throw your blood glucose out of control. It's important to have a plan in place before you become unwell, not when you can't think straight. Here's a general plan that should help; ask your health professionals if there is anything else you should do.

Know when to get help. Contact a health professional (for example, your GP, practice nurse or diabetes specialist nurse) if your illness continues for more than two days and you cannot eat or drink normally, if you are constantly vomiting and/or have diarrhoea, if your blood glucose level is consistently above 12mmol/l or if you have a high temperature that does not go down with your usual remedies.

Continue all your medications. Some people make the mistake of stopping their medications or insulin when they are so unwell that they don't feel like eating, but it is vital to keep taking all prescription drugs, especially because being unwell can raise your blood glucose. If you take insulin, your doctor may even suggest that you adjust (usually increase) the dosage when you are under the weather.

Check your blood glucose more frequently. When you start to feel unwell, your body goes on the defensive, sending out hormones to fight the illness. This is good news, of course, but the battle your body fights can raise your blood glucose and reduce your body's ability to use insulin. Usually your health professional will recommend that you check your blood glucose every 3 to 4 hours when you are feeling poorly, but be sure to discuss any specific recommendations before you become unwell. If your blood glucose readings are high when you are unwell, your health professional may recommend extra insulin.

Ask your health professional about checking your ketones. When you're unwell, if your blood glucose levels are consistently above 15mmol/l and you have Type 1 diabetes, you'll want to do a urine ketone test (available on prescription) to check for diabetic ketoacidosis, in which the body resorts to breaking down fat for energy and releases ketones, which poison the blood. This can happen if you have an infection, your blood glucose levels spiral out of control and you are very dehydrated through vomiting or diarrhoea or simply not being well enough to drink. The condition can become very serious. Signs of ketoacidosis are nausea, extreme thirst or dry

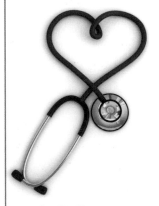

PLUS POINT
Being unwell can raise your blood glucose, so you will need to check your levels more often.

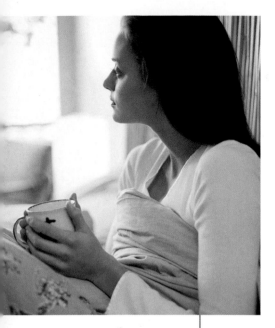

mouth, stomach pain, vomiting, blurred vision, flushed skin or fever, trouble breathing or paying attention, weakness or drowsiness, loss of appetite and a peardrop-smelling breath odour. If your ketone levels are high, get in touch with your GP immediately or go to A&E at a nearby hospital.

Keep sick day foods in the cupboard. You may not have much of an appetite when you are unwell, but it is important to eat as regularly as possible to help your blood glucose stay level. Try to choose foods from your normal healthy diet that are easy on the stomach such as soup, porridge, milkshakes and toast. Keep a supply of foods that might tempt your appetite when you are ill such as crispbreads, ice cream or fruit yoghurts.

Drink at least a mug of fluid every hour. When your blood glucose is high, your body tries to flush glucose out of your system by making you urinate more. This puts you at risk of dehydration; that's why increasing your fluid intake is crucial if you're not feeling well. If you can't keep food down, make up for that calorie loss by drinking sugary, caffeine-free fluids such as fruit juice, glucose drinks and non-diet soft drinks. Get medical help if you're showing symptoms of dehydration, including dry mouth, dry skin, cracked lips, extreme thirst, mental confusion and sunken eyes.

Get plenty of rest. It's true that physical activity will lower your blood glucose, but it isn't safe to exercise when you are unwell. It's more important to rest to allow your immune system to work on making you better. If you are restless, dim the light in your room by drawing the curtains, ask your partner or friend to rent a DVD for you, or listen to some relaxing music.

Before you become unwell, arrange for back-up help. When you're flat on your back with flu and trying to manage your diabetes, you probably won't have much energy left to run your household. Before you are laid low by illness, put plans in place to get the help you need. If you have children, call a relative or the parents of your children's closest friends and ask if they'd be willing to take care of them (offer to reciprocate where appropriate). Ask your partner to take over chores when you're feeling ill. Most important of all, find out exactly what you need to do to care for your diabetes when you're unwell. Diabetes UK has an information leaflet specifically about diabetes and illness, which you can get from the website or by contacting the Diabetes UK Careline (see details on page 271).

Tried-and-tested paths to effective weight loss

Most people with Type 2 diabetes struggle with their weight. And the chances are, you haven't been given much specific advice about losing pounds. But doing so is likely to make your blood glucose easier to control and can lower your blood pressure and cholesterol. If you lose a significant amount of weight you may be able to cut back on – or eliminate – some of your medications. The best way to get the weight off? Steer clear of the latest fad diet and stick to proven strategies.

Set moderate, achievable weight-loss goals. Research suggests that most people think they have to lose 3 to 7 stone (19kg to 44kg) to be 'successful' at weight loss – a belief that sets them up for failure. Instead, start with a reasonable goal, like losing 10lb (4.5kg). That kind of moderate weight loss still has a beneficial effect on diabetes – and if you reach that goal, you'll have the drive to lose another 10lb.

Know your BMI (Body Mass Index). To find out whether your body weight falls within the range of normal, overweight or obese, consult a BMI table or an online BMI calculator. If you're good with numbers, whip out a pencil and paper and run through the formula presented on page 254 (see Calculating your Body Mass Index). If your BMI is less than 25, your weight is normal. If your BMI is at least 25 but less than 30, you're overweight. If your BMI is 30 or above, you're considered obese.

Find a weight-loss partner. Dieting with a friend provides more than support – it can help you to lose more weight. That's what a recent Brown University, USA study of 109 people and their dieting partners found. Those with a motivated friend lost nearly twice as much weight as those who dieted on their own. Having someone within walking distance can be an added bonus. Find three friends who live nearby and announce your weight-loss intentions. The chances are they'll come on board as they have some weight to lose as well.

make the change

The habit: Losing 10-15lb (4.5-6.75kg).

The result: Improving your chances of preventing diabetes or related problems.

The evidence: In a major US research study called the Diabetes Prevention Program, people with prediabetes were given instructions to lose 7 per cent of their body weight (for an 11 stone/70kg person, that's 10½lb/4.7kg) through diet and exercise and to keep the weight off for the duration of the three-year study. Their risk of developing Type 2 diabetes dropped by 58 per cent. The lifestyle changes worked particularly well for people age 60 and older, reducing their risk by 71 per cent. If you already have diabetes, reducing your body weight by 5 to 7 per cent can improve your insulin sensitivity, which in turn lowers blood glucose. It can also lower your cholesterol and blood pressure.

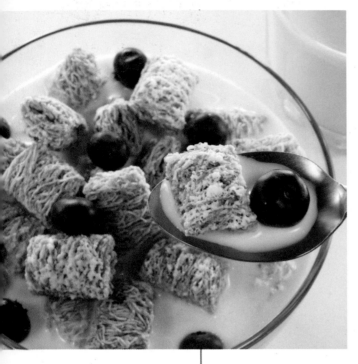

Join a weight-loss group. Research has consistently found that people who attend weight loss groups, join organisations or take courses lose more weight than those who diet independently. Ask about local groups or look online. There are lots of opportunities to 'share the experience' with others in the same boat and you can be confident that it will work.

Pair calorie-cutting with exercise. People who take more exercise while they are cutting calories tend to have an easier time losing weight and keeping it off than people who just cut calories. Burning an extra 250kcal a day – about the amount used in a brisk 45-minute walk – lops off about 26lb (11.7kg) a year, as long as you don't replace those calories with food.

Eat breakfast. Fibre helps you stay full, and a good way to get a healthy amount is to eat a breakfast cereal that contains at least 5g of fibre per serving. Breakfast does more than provide fibre, though. Studies show that eating breakfast helps you to eat less food later in the day – and consume fewer total calories.

Aim to lose weight slowly. You can shed just 1lb (0.5kg) a week – or even 2lb (1kg) a month – with small adjustments in your eating and physical activity. Don't let fad diet advertisements dazzle you with 'miracle' plans in which you can lose several stones in two months. Researchers say that people who achieve weight loss with such a diet typically put back most or all of the weight within five years. You're far better off learning how to make the lifestyle changes that will keep the weight off permanently, even if it means slower weight loss. What's more, crash diets that deprive you of essential nutrients can be very

Calculating your BMI (Body Mass Index)

To calculate your BMI, first square (multiply by itself) your height in metres. Then take your weight in kilograms and divide it by this figure. For example, suppose you weigh 75kg and your height is 1.67m. First square your height: 1.67 x 1.67 = 2.78 (rounded to 2.8). Now calculate your BMI: 75 divided by 2.8 = 26.98 (27).

dangerous. If you need guidance, there is plenty of support available through your surgery or clinic as well as from independent organisations. For example, Diabetes UK provides a great deal of information to get you started.

Ask your dietitian to design an individualised eating plan. It may not even seem like a weight-loss plan if your dietitian manages to integrate some of your favourite foods. A dietitian is trained to help you set reasonable calorie goals and make sure that your diet supplies the vitamins and minerals you need to help you manage your diabetes.

Keep a food diary for five days. Log everything you eat and drink, even if it's just water, a taste of ice cream or a breath mint. Your entries should include the time of day, size and number of servings, calories (a calorie-counting paperback book will help), what emotions you were feeling at the time and anything else that happened just before you ate. Food diaries are eye-openers for many people because so many of us eat without thinking about it. Review your food diary with a health professional you are working with, such as a dietitian, who will help you to identify situations or emotions that may cause you to overeat. These diaries can also be great tools for managing diabetes because they'll help you to remember what you ate that sent your blood glucose soaring, and what keeps your blood glucose on an even keel.

Consider bariatric surgery as a last resort. So-called 'stomach-stapling' surgery can have dramatically positive effects on some people's diabetes, practically reversing the condition. But don't take gastric bypass lightly; it's major surgery, so it's not without risks, including a 1 per cent risk of death from the surgery itself. Weight-loss surgery is recommended only for people who are severely obese and can't lose weight any other way. Those who have surgery have to commit to serious lifestyle changes: they will only be able to eat small meals, may need dietary supplements and perhaps medications, and will require frequent medical checkups. The cost of this surgery is substantial, too, and it is not generally available on the NHS.

whip it together!

Blueberry yoghurt surprise

Starting your morning with a delicious and healthy breakfast can keep you on track – eating well all day long. This sweet, crunchy yoghurt does the trick.

Add ½ teaspoon **sugar substitute** and 2 teaspoons **orange juice** to 75g **blueberries**. Let stand for 15 minutes. In a tall glass, make a layer of 8 tablespoons low-fat **Greek yoghurt** (if unavailable, use plain yoghurt and pour off excess water), ½ teaspoon lightly ground **linseeds**, and a quarter of the blueberries. Repeat the layers until all ingredients are used up.

Stamp out your cigarette addiction

Here's an ugly statistic: smoking adds a 12-fold increased risk of neuropathy, which is one of the main reasons for foot and leg amputation. If you're a smoker with diabetes, giving up should be your top priority. Diabetes is already putting your heart and blood vessels at risk, and the last thing you need is added damage from cigarettes. Smoking narrows your blood vessels, which can damage your heart; in some cases, it can lead to impotence and foot amputation. As someone with diabetes, you're already at high risk of developing kidney disease, nerve damage and eye damage; smoking increases your chances of developing all three.

Decide why you want to give up. About 70 per cent of people who smoke say they want to stop. But tobacco is addictive, there's no two ways about it. So for most people, giving up isn't easy. If better health isn't motivation enough, think about stopping for the sake of your loved ones. Whom will you miss, or who will miss you, if you die more than a decade prematurely? Stop smoking for them.

Stick motivational photos on the fridge. Want to be around for your granddaughter's wedding in 20 years? Put her smiling face on your fridge. Looking forward to retiring with your partner and driving through Europe? Get a magazine and cut out a picture of somewhere you want to visit, stick it up somewhere you'll see it often and imagine yourself there every day.

Work out when and why you smoke. Keep a list of the times of day and situations in which you're most likely to light up.

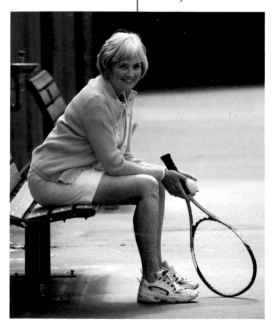

Understanding when you most 'need' a cigarette will help you devise things to do instead of smoking. If you need to have something to do with your hands while talking on the phone, fiddle with a pen or a small paperweight. If you like a cigarette with your morning coffee, start drinking tea instead. If a smoking break at work gives you an energy boost, go for a brisk walk around the car park instead .

Exercise regularly. It can help you to stop smoking by burning off stress hormones so you feel less of an urge to smoke and by producing feel-good brain chemicals to help reduce the uncomfortable effects of nicotine withdrawal. A Gallup Poll found that smokers who exercised were twice as likely to give up as their sedentary counterparts. Daily exercise can also help you to avoid the dreaded 5–10lb (2.25–4.5kg) weight gain commonly associated with kicking the habit.

Tell everyone you know that you're giving up. When your family, friends and colleagues all know you are trying to give up cigarettes, they'll provide encouragement and will be less likely to put temptation in your path. And when you know that you're accountable to everyone around you, you will be less likely to cheat and sneak away for a crafty puff.

Give yourself a smoke-free deadline. Pick a date in the near future when you're pretty sure that you won't have any major stressful issues to deal with. If your daughter is getting married in three weeks, or if you're moving house, changing jobs or hosting a big party soon, put off your deadline until after the chaos has died down. The more stressed you are, the stronger your cravings (and withdrawal symptoms) are likely to be.

Choose the cessation method that will work best for you. If you're a casual smoker, you may be able to just go cold turkey. But if you're a heavy smoker, you will probably need to wean yourself off nicotine by means of nicotine patches or chewing gum or by using nasal sprays or inhalers. (Some of these treatments are available over-the-counter and some are available on prescription.) If you're comfortable with alternative treatments, hypnosis and acupuncture may be worth looking into. Your clinic, surgery and pharmacy all have information and support to help you choose what will work for you.

If you use patches, keep an eye on your blood glucose. Nicotine patches can raise glucose levels; you'll want to check your blood glucose more frequently than you typically do so that you get a good sense of how the patch affects you. And never smoke while you're on nicotine patches – nicotine can be toxic in large doses, and the combination of patch and tobacco could be deadly.

Throw away your smoking paraphernalia. When you don't have ashtrays, lighters and other tobacco-related accessories in your home, it will be more difficult for you to light up on impulse.

Have your curtains, clothes and rugs cleaned professionally. Do whatever it takes to banish the stale-smoke smell that your home might have. Smoke permeates just about every kind of fabric; if you smoke indoors, the chances are your home smells stale, and you're so used to it that you don't even notice the odour. Once all your soft furnishings have been professionally cleaned, you'll

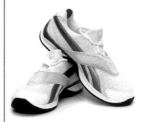

PLUS POINT
Exercise can help to motivate your bid to quit. Smokers who exercise are twice as likely to be able to kick the addiction.

see how fresh 'smoke-free' living can smell. And remembering all the money you've just spent to get everything clean might just keep you from reaching for another cigarette.

Make your home a no-smoking zone. Post 'no smoking' signs, banish ashtrays and make it clear to anyone who visits your home that they shouldn't light up under your roof. It's your house and if you have made the commitment not to smoke, no one else should be allowed to smoke on your premises, either!

Create diversions. Smoking is a pastime as much as it is an addiction. You smoke for something to do during breaks at work, while driving your car and during quiet evenings at home. Once you give up, you'll feel that something is missing during these times. Fill the space with other activities. Sing along to a favourite CD while you drive. Take short walks instead of coffee breaks. Choose hands-on activities such as crosswords or jigsaws as you wind down in the evening. You'll miss cigarettes less if you keep busy.

Take 10. When the urge to light up strikes, look at your watch and give yourself 10 minutes. During that time take full, deep breaths as you would if you were drawing on a cigarette. Deep breathing will fill your lungs with clean, smoke-free air and trigger a relaxation response. By the time 10 minutes is up, the acute urge to smoke will have passed and you'll be able to move past the craving.

Join a stop-smoking group. This may be just the ticket if you need support in banishing tobacco from your life. You may find there is a group at your surgery, diabetes clinic or at work. Alternatively, you may source groups through local papers and via the internet. Heart, cancer and diabetes organisations also run such groups.

If you relapse, try again ... and again. Don't give up on giving up. Most people have to try to kick the habit several times before they're finally successful. Your first three smoke-free months will be the hardest. While you are battling cravings, remind yourself that doing without tobacco won't always be this uncomfortable or difficult. In the meantime, avoid alcohol, which will lower your resolve, and avoid other people who are smoking.

Get away from secondhand smoke, too. Being in the company of smokers not only tempts fate, it also hurts your heart. Persistent exposure to cigarette smoke, at home or at work, nearly doubles your risk of having a heart attack even if you don't smoke, according to a ten-year study of more than 32,000 women. If you socialise with smokers, do so in places where they can puff outdoors. If you live with a smoker, take the ashtray outside and keep it there.

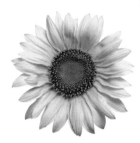

PLUS POINT
Don't give up. Most people have to try to stop smoking several times before they are successful.

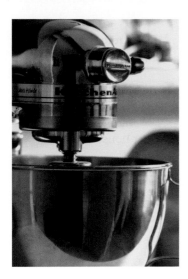

16
Tools

Staying on top of your diabetes means

staying on top of your meals, your

medication, your blood glucose levels,

your clinic appointments and more.

Use these handy tools and resources

to make living healthily a little easier.

My medication record

Name:

What it's for:

Amount: How often:

When to take:

Name:

What it's for:

Amount: How often:

When to take:

Name:

What it's for:

Amount: How often:

When to take:

Name:

What it's for:

Amount: How often:

When to take:

Name:

What it's for:

Amount: How often:

When to take:

Name:

What it's for:

Amount: How often:

When to take:

Name:

What it's for:

Amount: How often:

When to take:

My daily food and exercise log

Use this chart for a more detailed look at how your meals and physical activity affect your blood glucose. If cutting portion sizes and carbohydrates at one meal still leaves your blood glucose high before the next meal, try adding exercise to bring the levels down.

Day:_____ **Date:**_____

morning
Breakfast Time: _____ Blood glucose before eating: _____

ITEM	AMOUNT	CARBS*

Blood glucose 2 hours after eating: _____

Snack Time: _____

ITEM	AMOUNT	CARBS*

Exercise Time: _____

ACTIVITY _____

DURATION _____

midday
Breakfast Time: _____ Blood glucose before eating: _____

ITEM	AMOUNT	CARBS*

Blood glucose 2 hours after eating: _____

Snack Time: _____

ITEM	AMOUNT	CARBS*

Exercise Time: _____

ACTIVITY _____

DURATION _____

evening
Breakfast Time: _____ Blood glucose before eating: _____

ITEM	AMOUNT	CARBS*

Blood glucose 2 hours after eating: _____

Snack Time: _____

ITEM	AMOUNT	CARBS*

Exercise Time: _____

ACTIVITY _____

DURATION _____

*portions or grams.

Common foods and their glycaemic loads

The glycaemic load (GL) is a measure of how much a serving of a particular food raises a person's blood glucose. Your own reaction might be somewhat different, so it's best to check your blood glucose 2 hours after eating a food to find out how it has been affected. We've grouped foods into three categories: low GL (10 or under), medium GL (11 to 19) and high GL (20 or higher). The higher the GL, the more the food will raise your blood glucose. The GL is closely tied to portion size; if you eat twice as much as the portion size indicated, the food will have double the effect on your blood glucose.

Low (GL = 10 or under)

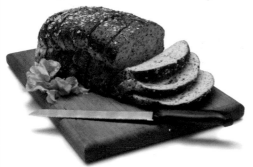

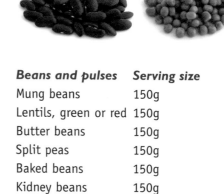

Breads	Serving size	GL
Rye bread	30g	5
Mixed grain bread	1 slice (30g)	6
Wheat tortilla	2 x 15cm	6
Wholemeal bread	1 slice (30g)	8
Ryvita crispbread	25g	9
White bread	1 slice (30g)	10
Gluten free multigrain	1 slice (30g)	10
Pitta bread (white)	1 medium (30g)	10

Beans and pulses	Serving size	GL
Mung beans	150g	4
Lentils, green or red	150g	5
Butter beans	150g	6
Split peas	150g	6
Baked beans	150g	7
Kidney beans	150g	7
Chickpeas	150g	8
Lima beans	150g	10

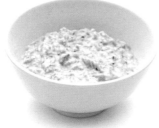

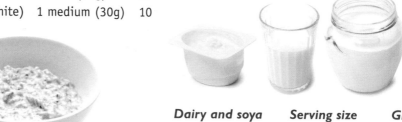

Breakfast cereals	Serving size	GL
Porridge (cooked)	250g	9
All-Bran	30g	9
Alpen Muesli	30g	10

Dairy and soya	Serving size	GL
Milk	250ml	3
Reduced fat ice cream	50g	5
Soya milk	250ml	8
Low-fat yoghurt with fruit and sugar	200ml	9

Low (GL = 10 or under) continue

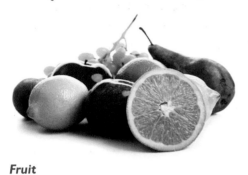

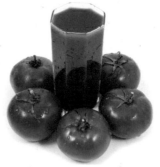

Fruit and vegetables	Serving size	GL
Cherries	about 16 (120g)	3
Grapefruit	½	3
Carrot, raw	1 large	3
Pear	1 small	4
Strawberries	about 6 medium	4
Watermelon	120g	4
Beetroot	80g	5
Orange	1 small	5
Peach	1 small	5
Plums	2 small	5
Apple	1 small	6
Kiwi fruit	120g	6
Pineapple	120g	7
Swede	150g	7
Sweetcorn	80g	7
Grapes	small bunch	8
Mango	120g	8
Apricots, dried	60g	9
Paw paw	120g	10
Prunes	60g	10

Drinks	Serving size	GL
Tomato juice	250ml	4
Grapefruit juice, unsweetened	250ml	7

Sweets and snacks	Serving size	GL
Nutella (chocolate hazelnut spread)	20g	4
M&Ms with peanuts	small packet (30g)	6
Popcorn	20g	8
Scone	1 small (25g)	8

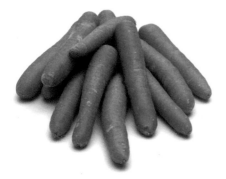

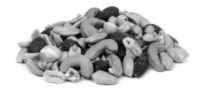

Nuts	Serving size	GL
Peanuts	45g	1
Cashew nuts	about 13 (45g)	3
Mixed nuts, roasted	45g	4

Medium (GL = 11–19)

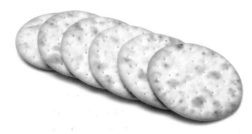

Breads, crisps and crackers

Breads, crisps and crackers	Serving size	GL
Gluten-free white bread	1 slice (30g)	11
Turkish bread	30g	15
White baguette	30g	15
Pretzels	30g	16
Corn crisps	50g	17
Rice cakes	25g	17

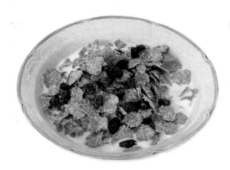

Breakfast Cereals	Serving size	GL
Raisin Bran	30g	12
Weetabix	30g	13
Frosties	30g	15
Shredded Wheat	30g	15
Golden Grahams	30g	18

Grains	Serving size	GL
Pearl barley	150g (cooked)	11
Bulghur wheat	150g (cooked)	12
Brown rice	150g (cooked)	18
Quinoa	150g (cooked)	18
Wild rice	150g (cooked)	18

Pasta	Serving size	GL
Whole-wheat spaghetti	180g (cooked)	13
White spaghetti	180g (cooked)	18
Fettucine	180g (cooked)	18

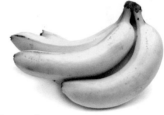

Fruits and Vegetables	Serving size	GL
Banana	120g	12
Figs	60g	16
Parsnips	80g	12
Mashed potato	150g	15
Boiled potato	150g	17
Sweet potato	150g	17

Beans and Pulses	Serving size	GL
Haricot beans	150g	12
Black-eyed beans	150g	13

Drinks	Serving size	GL
Apple juice	250ml	12
Orange juice	250ml	13
Pineapple juice	250ml	16
Cranberry juice	250ml	16

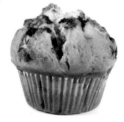

Sweets and snacks	Serving size	GL
Sponge cake	1 slice	17
Doughnut	1 small	17
Blueberry muffin	1 medium	17
Twix	1 (60g)	17

High (GL = 20 or higher)

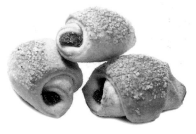

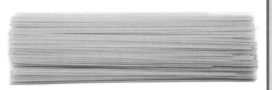

Breads	Serving size	GL
Chapatti	1 (60g)	21
Hamburger roll	1	21
Pain au chocolat	1 (70g)	27
Middle Eastern flatbread	1 large	30

Pasta	Serving size	GL
Linguini	180g (cooked)	22
Macaroni	180g (cooked)	23
Udon noodles	180g (cooked)	26

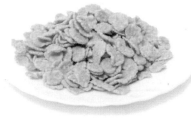

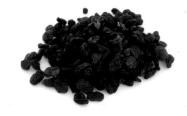

Breakfast Cereals	Serving size	GL
Cornflakes	30g	20
Special K	30g	20
Rice Krispies	30g	21
Pop Tarts	50g	25

Dried Fruit	Serving size	GL
Dates	60g	25
Sultanas	60g	25
Raisins	60g	28

Drinks	Serving size	GL
Lucozade	250ml	40
Orange fizzy drink	250ml	23

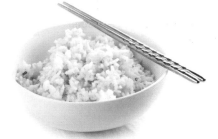

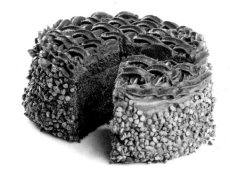

Grains	Serving size	GL
Basmati rice	150g (cooked)	23
Couscous	150g (cooked)	23
Long-grain white rice	150g (cooked)	23
Sticky white rice	150g (cooked)	31

Sweets	Serving size	GL
Chocolate cake	100g	20
Jelly beans	30g	22
Mars Bar	1 (60g)	26

Source: www.mendosa.com/gilists.htm

Carbohydrate exchanges

One good way to keep your blood glucose under control is to eat approximately the same amount of carbohydrate every day and distribute those carbs fairly evenly throughout the day. Carbohydrate counting helps you do it. Start by knowing how many grams of carbs/carb portions' you should eat each day (see page 53), then use this list as a handy reference. Each food listed below, in the amount specified, equals approximately 10g of carbohydrate (one carb portion) unless otherwise noted. The foods will vary in the number of calories they contain based on their fat and protein content.

Breads
1 small slice
½ wholemeal bap
3cm slice of French bread
1 small crumpet
15cm tortilla
¼ bagel
½ croissant
2 cracker breads

Cereals
3 tbsp All Bran
2 tbsp branflakes
2½ tbsp cornflakes
1 Weetabix
20g uncooked rolled oats
3 tbsp Special K
2 tbsp Fruit 'n Fibre

Pastas and grains
1 tbsp brown or white rice
2 tbsp pasta
1 sheet lasagna
1 tbsp couscous

Biscuits
1 digestive
2 Rich Tea
2 Garibaldi
1 small cookie

Snacks
1 small packet crisps
100g peanuts
50g cashew nuts
30g bag Bombay mix
2 cream crackers
½ cereal bar

Fruits
1 small apple
4 dried apricots
½ medium banana
10 grapes
1 grapefruit
2 kiwi fruits
⅓ mango
1 slice of melon
1 medium orange
1 medium peach
1 small pear
1 slice of fresh pineapple
2 plums
3 dried prunes
15 strawberries

Dairy foods
200ml (⅓ pint) milk
1 small pot of yoghurt
1 tbsp custard powder
1 small scoop of dairy ice
  cream

Vegetables & potatoes
2 tbsp baked beans
2 tbsp kidney beans
2 tbsp chickpeas
1 egg-sized boiled potato
5 medium-cut chips
1 scoop mashed potato
¼ large baked potato
2 tbsp peas
1½ tbsp sweetcorn

Sweets & cakes (with 30g-40g carbohydrate – 3 or 4 carb portions)
1 doughnut
1 flapjack
1 small chocolate éclair
Cadbury's dairy milk
  chocolate bar (49g)
4-finger Kit Kat

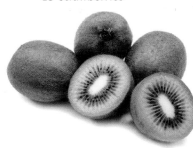

Shopping list

If you're planning your meals as we suggest, create a shopping list based on the recipes on the week's menus. Here's a list of healthy staples to get you started. Remember our tip to fill up to half your shopping trolley with colourful fresh produce.

Fresh foods

Fruit
- Berries
- Apples
- Bananas
- Oranges or grapefruit
- Nectarines or peaches
- Mangoes
- Kiwi fruit
- Cantaloupe

Protein foods
- Fresh fish or seafood
- Chicken breast
- Lean beef (limit red meat to two servings per week)
- Turkey or chicken breast from the deli counter
- Eggs

Vegetables
- Broccoli
- Spinach
- Tomatoes (include cherry tomatoes for munching)
- Carrots (including baby carrots for munching)
- Shredded carrots for salads
- Avocado
- Lettuce (not iceberg)
- Cabbage or bok choy
- Red, yellow or green peppers
- Garlic
- Onions
- Cauliflower for 'cauliflower rice' (page 61)
- Your vegetable of the week

Dairy counter
- Skimmed milk
- Evaporated semi-skimmed milk
- Plain low-fat yoghurt
- Low-fat cheddar cheese
- Low-fat mini cheeses
- Feta cheese
- Soya milk
- Margarine (free of trans fats)

Other
- Linseeds, whole
- Mustard
- Meal replacement drinks such as Slimfast
- Hummus (not with tahini)
- Fresh tomato salsa

Storecupboard foods

Grains
- 100% wholemeal bread
- Whole-wheat tortillas
- Whole-wheat pasta
- Barley
- Brown rice
- Old-fashioned porridge oats
- Couscous (preferably whole-wheat)
- Cereals with at least 5g of fibre per serving

Tinned Foods
- Oily fish such as sardines
- Salmon

- Black, kidney and pinto beans

Spices
- Basil
- Cayenne pepper
- Cinnamon
- Dry rubs for meats
- Ginger
- Italian seasoning
- Lemon-herb seasoning
- Oregano
- Rosemary
- Turmeric (or curry powder)

Other
- Extra-virgin olive oil
- Linseed oil
- Rapeseed oil
- Walnut oil
- Natural peanut butter
- Cereal bars with at least 6g of fibre and no more than 100kcal per bar
- Crispbreads or oatcakes
- Unsalted nuts
- Tea bags
- Sea salt

For the freezer
- Frozen berries
- Frozen broccoli florets, carrots or mixed vegetables
- Frozen chicken mini fillets

- Frozen soya beans
- Frozen fish that has been sustainably caught (plain not breaded or battered)
- Frozen prawns

- Frozen chocolate milk sticks (less than 80kcal each)

Sample meal plans

The following menus are examples of just how easy it is to get plenty of fruit and vegetables into your meals while keeping calories and carbohydrates under control. Each menu contains approximately 1,600 to 1,800kcal; if you need fewer or more calories per day, you'll need to adjust portion sizes accordingly. Consult your dietitian to discuss how these menus might fit into your own eating plan.

Easy weekday menu

During the week, everything is a routine. But it needn't be boring. Here's an easy, delicious menu for those busy days.

Breakfast
- 30g high-fibre cereal (5g or more per serving)
- Half a pint of semi-skimmed milk
- Handful fresh blueberries

Lunch
- Cranberry turkey sandwich:
  75g lean turkey breast, 1 sliced tomato, salad leaves, half a grated carrot, 1 tsp cranberry sauce, 2 medium slices wholemeal bread
- Quarter of a cucumber, sliced, and 7 cherry tomatoes, drizzled with 1 tsp olive oil and 1 tsp balsamic vinegar
- 1 Granny Smith apple

Dinner
- 125g grilled sustainably caught white fish with 2 tbsp **Tropical fruit salsa** (page 51)
- 3 tbsp **Garlicky green beans** (page 49)
- 4 tbsp steamed brown rice
- Small bowl tossed green salad with 2 tbsp fat-free Italian dressing

Snacks
- 1 low-fat mini cheese or 1 cereal bar (less than 100kcal)
- 1 serving (4 crisps) **Crispy cheese crisps** page 66)

On the go

One look at your 'to-do' list and you know you are going to have a hectic day. Just be prepared with this on-the-go menu that even incorporates a ready-made lunch.

Breakfast
- 1 serving Blueberry yoghurt surprise (page 255) prepared in a lock-top box
- Half a whole-grain roll spread with 2 tsp peanut butter

Lunch
- 1 small plain hamburger from a fast-food outlet
- Side salad with low-fat dressing
- 1 small apple

Dinner
- 1 serving **Cook-and-freeze turkey rice casserole** (page 41)
- Small bowl green salad with 1 tsp olive oil and 2 tsp red wine vinegar
- 80g fresh pineapple chunks

Snacks
- 1 serving **Garlic roasted soya beans** (page 206)
- 1 small banana

Weekend

Aaah. The weekend. You've looked forward all week long to putting up your feet and relaxing a bit. Since you have more free time at the weekend, spend some of it in the kitchen whipping up a delectable meal. These menu suggestions require not much more than one pan and just a few extra minutes in the kitchen.

Breakfast
- Omelette: 2 eggs mixed with a splash of semi-skimmed milk, with half a chopped red pepper and a quarter of an onion (chopped), cooked in a nonstick pan with 1 tsp olive oil
- 1 medium slice wholemeal toast with 1 tsp pure fruit spread
- 8 sliced strawberries

Lunch
- Sweet curried chicken salad sandwich: 75–100g cooked diced white chicken, half an apple (grated), half a carrot (grated), and 1 tbsp low-fat mayonnaise mixed with 2 tsp honey, 1 tsp curry powder, served in 1–2 wholemeal pitta breads and topped with shredded lettuce

- 1 carrot cut into sticks
- 10 red grapes

Dinner
- 1 serving **Balsamic mustard-grilled prawn kebabs** (page 99)
- 50g uncooked weight bulghur wheat (cooked according to pack instructions and served under the prawns)
- 1 serving **Apple coleslaw** (page 97)

Snacks
- 1 serving **Double-rich chocolate pudding treat** (page 246)
- 1 small peach

Entertaining

Everyone will enjoy this special menu whether they have diabetes or not. Your guests will look forward to coming back and enjoying your cooking very soon.

Breakfast
- 3 mini breakfast pancakes (shop-bought or homemade)
- 2 tsp honey
- 2 handfuls raspberries
- 200ml semi-skimmed milk (to drink)

Lunch
- 1 serving **Pearl barley and chickpea salad** (page 21)
- Small bowl romaine lettuce tossed with a quarter of a cucumber (diced) and half a carrot (grated) with 1 tsp walnut oil and 2 tsp cider vinegar
- 1 small nectarine

Dinner
- 1 serving **Seared white fish in zesty herb and tomato sauce** (page 224)
- 3 tbsp steamed broccoli
- 1 serving straight-to-wok or egg noodles

Snacks
- 1 serving **Sweet balsamic onion hummus** (page 70) with 2–3 crispbreads
- Quarter of a mango, sliced and sprinkled with 1 tsp lime juice

Know your numbers : recommended target levels

Use this table to monitor your results against those recommended or your personal targets, to see your progress towards them.

Test	Recommended healthy level*	Your personal Target**	Your level (date)	Your level (date)	Your level (date)
Blood glucose fasting 2 hours after a meal	4-6 mmol/l less than 10 mmol/l				
HbA1c	6.5% or less 6.5-7.5% if you are prone to severe hypoglycaemia				
Blood pressure	130/80mmHg or less				
Waist size Women Asian men Black and white Men	Less than 80cm Less than 90cm Less than 94cm				
Body mass index	20–25				
Total cholesterol	4mmol/l or less				
HDL cholesterol Women Men	1.2mmol/l or more 1.0mmol/l or more				
Triglycerides	Less than 1.7mmol/l				

*These levels are based on current national guidance.

**Your personal target level may vary from this, according to discussion with, and recommendation from your health professional.

Organisations and resources

British Association for Counselling and Psychotherapy
BACP House, 15 St John's Business Park,
Lutterworth LE17 4HB
Tel 01455 883300
www.bacp.co.uk

British Heart Foundation
14 Fitzhardinge Street,
London W1H 6DH
Tel 020 7935 0185
Helpline 0845 070 80 70 (Mon-Fri, 9am–5pm)
www.bhf.org.uk

Diabetes UK
Macleod House, 10 Parkway,
London NW1 7AA
Tel 020 7424 1000
Careline 0845 120 2960 (Mon-Fri, 9am–5pm)
www.diabetes.org.uk

Juvenile Diabetes Research Foundation
19 Angel Gate, City Road,
London EC1V 2PT
Tel 020 7713 2030
www.jdrf.org.uk

MedicAlert Foundation
1 Bridge Wharf,
156 Caledonian Road,
London N1 9UU
Tel 0207 833 3034
Helpline 0800 581420 (Mon-Fri, 9am–5pm)
www.medicalert.org.uk

Royal National Institute for the Blind
105 Judd Street,
London WC1H 9NE
Tel 0207 388 1266
Helpline 0845 766 9999 (Mon-Fri, 9am–5pm)
www.rnib.org.uk

Samaritans
The Upper Mill,
Kingston Road,
Ewell,
Surrey, KT 17 2AF
www.samaritans.org
24 hour UK helpline: 08457 909090
email: jo@samaritans.org

The Sexual Dysfunction Association
Suite 301, Emblem House,
London Bridge Hospital,
27 Tooley Street, London SE1 2PR
Tel 0870 7743571
Helpline 0870 7743571 (Mon, Wed, Fri 10am–4pm).
www.impotence.org.uk

Successful Diabetes
PO Box 819, Northampton, NN4 4AG
08445 617205
www.successfuldiabetes.com
Offers a range of resources to help people with diabetes to manage their condition

The Stroke Association
Stroke House, 240 City Road,
London EC1V 2PR
Tel: 0207 566 0300
Helpline: 0845 303 3100 (Mon–Fri 9am–5pm)
www.stroke.org.uk

UK National Kidney Federation
The Point, Coach Road, Shireoaks,
Worksop, Nottinghamshire S81 8BW
Tel: 01909 544999
Helpline 0845 601 0209 (Mon–Fri, 9am–5pm)
www.kidney.org.uk

USEFUL WEBSITES
To contact others with diabetes:
www.diabetes-insight.info
www.insulin-pumpers.org.uk

For information about the Glycaemic Index:
www.glycaemicindex.com

The Department of Health
www.dh.gov.uk

To stop smoking:
http://gosmokefree.nhs.uk
Helpline 0800 022 4332 (Daily 7am–11pm)

www.quit.org.uk
UK Quitline 0800 002200 (Daily 9am–9pm)

Action on Smoking and Health
www.ash.org.uk

A

B

Beating Diabetes is published by The Reader's Digest Association Limited,
11 Westferry Circus, Canary Wharf, London E14 4HE

Beating Diabetes is adapted from *759 Secrets for beating diabetes* published by The Reader's Digest Association, Inc. in 2007.

We are committed both to the quality of our products and the service we provide to our customers. We value your comments, so please do contact us on **08705 113366** or via our website at **www.readersdigest.co.uk**

If you have any comments or suggestions about the content of our books, email us at **gbeditorial@readersdigest.co.uk**

Colour origination: Colour Systems Limited, London
Printed and bound in China

Reader's Digest Project Team
Project editor Rachel Warren Chadd
Assistant editor Celia Coyne
Art editor Simon Webb
Designer Keith Davis
Proofreader Ron Pankhurst
Indexer Marie Lorimer

Reader's Digest General Books
Editorial director Julian Browne
Art director Anne-Marie Bulat
Head of book development Sarah Bloxham
Managing editor Nina Hathway
Picture resource manager Christine Hinze
Pre-press account manager Dean Russell
Product production manager Claudette Bramble
Production controller Katherine Tibbals

ISBN: 978 0 276 44409 8
Concept code: US6007/IC
Book code: 400-403 UP0000-1
Oracle Code: 250013010S.00.24